PRASARA YOGA
Flow Beyond Thought

प्रसर

BY SCOTT SONNON

THE FLOW COACH™

PRASARA YOGA: *Flow Beyond Thought*

Copyright ©2007 by RMAX.tv Productions

All rights reserved. No part of this work may be reproduced or utilized in any form or by any means, electronic or mechanical, including photocopying, recording, or by any information storage and retrieval system, without the prior written permission of the publisher.

For information on Scott Sonnon and RMAX.tv Productions, please contact:
RMAX.tv Productions
P.O. Box 501388
Atlanta, GA 31150
Website: www.rmaxinternational.com

Comments and questions should be sent to: info@rmaxinternational.com

Circular Strength Training® and Clubbell® are registered trademarks of RMAX.tv Productions.

Printed and bound in the United States of America.

ISBN-13: 978-0-9794275-4-1
ISBN-10: 0-9794275-4-1

CREDITS

Editing: Amy Norcross

Design and Layout: Wade Munson • www.wadeincreativity.com

Photography: John Meloy • www.johnnydanger.net

Contributing Authors: Coach Ryan Hurst, CST3; Coach Jarlo Ilano, CST2; and Mushtaq Ali Al-Ansari, Ph.D.

Sanskrit Provided By: Mushtaq Ali Al-Ansari, Ph.D.

Photographic Model: Summer Huntington

DISCLAIMER

None of the information contained in this book is intended to be taken as medical advice. Should you have any condition that requires professional medical attention, please always consult a doctor before you begin any exercises presented in this book or any other source. Albeit the information and advice in this book are believed to be accurate, neither the publisher nor the author will be held liable for any injury, damages, losses, claims, actions, proceedings, expenses, or costs (including legal) that result from using instructions, advice, or exercises in this book.

PRASARA YOGA: *Flow Beyond Thought*

I walked backwards into yoga, and fell into the arms of the most beautiful person I have ever met, Sri Mata Amritanandamayi Devi (www.amma.org).

This book, everything I believe that I know, have yet to understand, and will strive my life in living up to in gratitude, I devote to her humanitarian efforts.

As Amma says, *"Where there is love, there is no effort."*

The physical discipline of yoga, Amma teaches, prepares us to serve others through love. If this book can help you make that preparation more useful and accessible, then I feel grateful.

In love and service,

Scott Sonnon

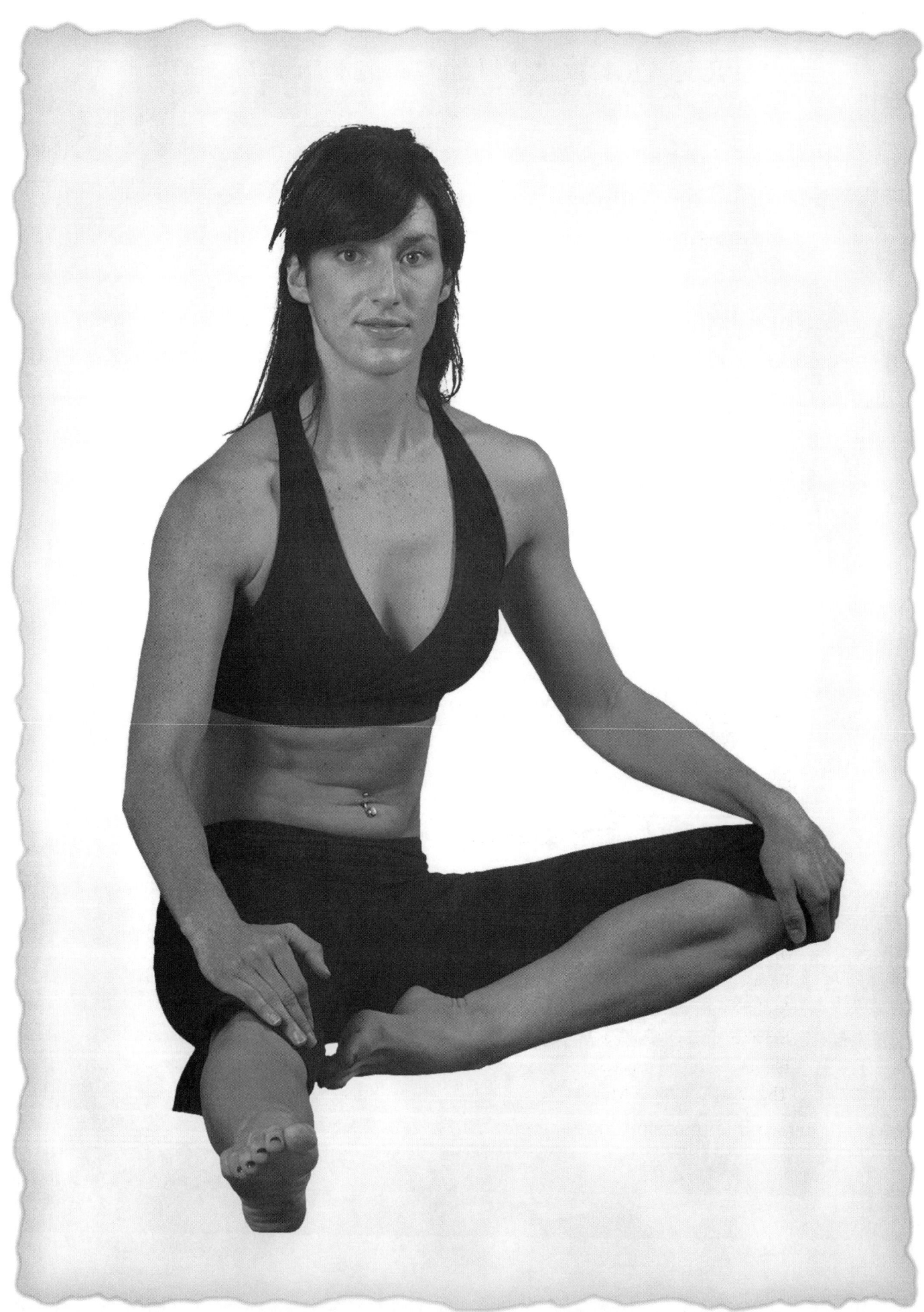

PRASARA YOGA: *Flow Beyond Thought*

TABLE OF CONTENTS

INTRODUCTION ix

PART ONE

RESEARCH IMPETUS 3
    Where's the Mind? 3
    Yoga That Isn't Fixed 4
    Zeno's Paradox: Infinite Digression and Movement Impossibility 4
    The Arrow Paradox 5
    No Abiding Place 6
    Ongoing Evolution 6
    Reclaiming the Personal Process 7

DEFINING PRASARA 9
    Prasara Yoga and the Spirit of Patanjali 9
    Vinyasa: The Art of Breath 9
    Prasara: The Art of Movement 10
    Flow: The Eighth Limb of Yoga 10

FINDING A BALANCED PERSPECTIVE OF HATHA YOGA 13

DEFINING ASANA IN EXERCISE PHYSIOLOGY 17
    Debunking the Stretching Myth 18
    Flexibility Versus Elasticity 19
    Stored Elastic Energy and Viscosity 19
    The Stretch Reflex 20
    Viscoelasticity: Flexibility Is Speed Specific 21
    Health Risks of Static Stretching 21
    Short-Range Stiffness 22
    Plasticity Changes 22
    Mobility — The Antiaging Agent 23
    Static Stretching Versus Asana 23
    Balance and Proprioception 24
    The Dysfunction of Mirrors 25

DEFINING BODY FLOW IN EXERCISE PHYSIOLOGY 29

PRASARA YOGA: *Flow Beyond Thought*

THE PROGRESSIVE DEGREES OF BODY FLOW......................................33
- Three Planes of Movement..33
- Three Axes of Rotation..34
- Six Degrees of Freedom..34
- Pain-Free Mobility: What Causes Pain?....................35
- Joint Nutrition...36
- Resolving Swelling..36
- Rehabilitation...36
- Chronic Pain Creates Fear-Reactivity..........................36
- Dynamic Mobility Training 37

DEFINING BOUND FLOW IN EXERCISE PHYSIOLOGY 39

THE PROGRESSIVE STAGES OF BOUND FLOW................................41

THE SITE IS NOT THE SOURCE 45

COMPENSATORY MOVEMENT..47
- We Are How and What We Move!.............................47
- Not Moving Is a Form of Moving!..............................48

THE BIOCHEMISTRY OF THE BODY FLOW 49

GOOD VIBRATIONS..53

WHAT IS FEAR-REACTIVITY?...57
- We Are Not Our Additions..57
- The Physical-to-Emotional-to-Mental Process 58

ADAPTATION AND PROGRESSION OF FEAR-REACTIVITY................61
- Stress Arousal Scale..61

TOLERANCE AFFECTS HEALTH, STRENGTH, AND PERFORMANCE...........63

THE STRESS AROUSAL SYNDROME 67

WHAT IS THE SIXTH SENSE?..71

WHAT IS PROPRIOCEPTION?...73

MENTAL BLUEPRINT AND SELF-IMAGE...75

THRESHOLD OF PAIN = THRESHOLD OF PERFORMANCE..............77

INTUITIVE PRACTICE 79
- The Peripheral Nervous System..................................79
- The Brain 80

INTUITIVE PRACTICE: GOING TO THE EDGE....................................83

PRASARA YOGA: *Flow Beyond Thought*

CALISTHENICS VERSUS YOGA 85
CORE ACTIVATION INSIDE OUT 87
    Inner to Outer Unit Core Activation 87
        What Is the Outer Unit? 87
        What Is the Inner Unit? 88
    Dangers of Fitness Core Training 88
    The Firing Sequence of Inner to Outer Unit 89
    Fitness Core Training Versus Core Activation 89
    Like a String of Pearls 91
SYNCING BREATH 93
    Breath Mastery Scale 94
    Depth of Breath 94
    Relationship Between Depth and Effort 95
PERPETUAL FLOW 97
    The Sun Salutation Example 98
        Finding a Match 98
        Hemming It Up 99
        Adding a Patch 99
    We Are Only in Transition from One Thing to the Next! 100
FROM RECOVERY TO COORDINATION TO REFINEMENT 101
DEVELOPING PROPER FORM 103
CONCLUSION 105

PART TWO

FOREST 109
SPIDER MONKEY 119
DIVING DOLPHIN 129
TUMBLEWEED 137
FLOCK OF PIGEONS 147

BIBLIOGRAPHY 159

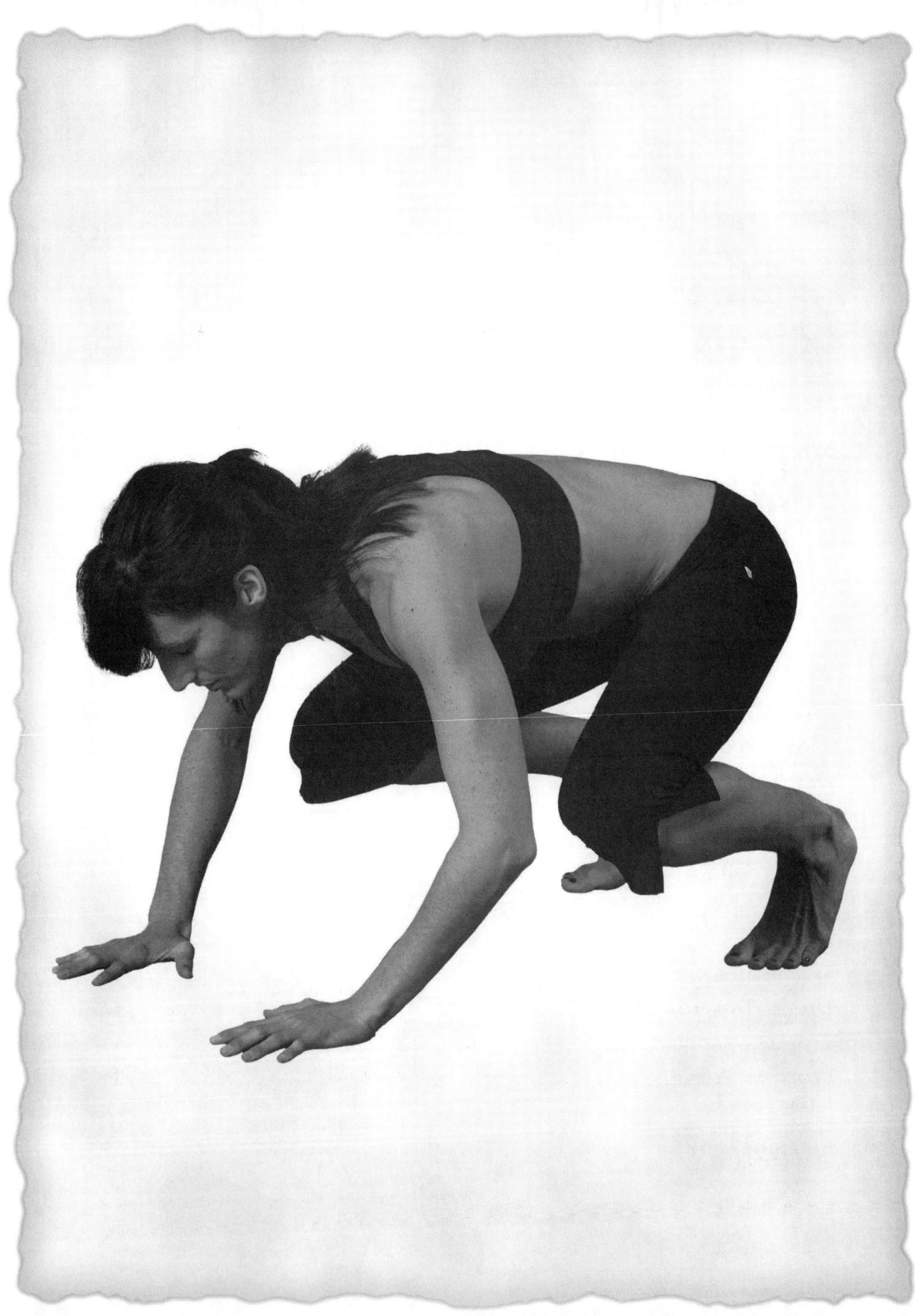

Introduction

I have been involved with physical activities since a very young age. I spent more than 10 years competing in gymnastics and have been involved with martial arts twice as long. While I was studying martial arts in Japan, a friend of mine first introduced me to yoga and the many health benefits that can be achieved through the daily study of it. I soon realized that yoga was a great way to help with the stress of daily life, especially while living in Japan. I religiously Down-Dogged myself into my yoga practice and found that the movements and breathing exercises really helped me clear my head after a long day of packed trains and fast-talking Osakans. That was a little more than eight years ago.

I continued with my daily practice, but it wasn't until I was introduced to Scott Sonnon that my physical, and especially mental, practice took on a completely new light.

The gymnastic-like movements of Prasara yoga brought me back to the times of when I was young, and I immediately fell in love with this "new" yoga. But you don't have to be a gymnast, a martial artist, or an athlete to fully receive the benefits of Prasara yoga.

When I first became involved with Prasara yoga I knew that it was something special. However, I didn't realize just what an impact it would have on the way I viewed my personal practice and how I now view yoga as a whole. What I thought was this new yoga called Prasara was actually the essence of what we are striving for in our own yoga. That essence is flow.

Yoga in Sanskrit means "to yoke" or "to join." Many yoga systems talk about joining the body with the mind and the breathing with the poses in order to attain flow. Yet what Prasara yoga shows is that there is one very important component that has been missing from Western yoga to attain flow. That component is including movement. Flow is not just where breathing and structure, the poses, merge. It is also the merging of the integral element of movement. Without the joined forces of these three — structure, breathing, and movement — you will not find your flow.

Finding your flow and learning how to apply it in your daily life are what this book is about.

PRASARA YOGA: *Flow Beyond Thought*

I'm truly honored to be able to write this foreword. I cannot express how profound and life changing Prasara yoga has been for me. I believe that you will find the same to be true with your own personal yoga practice in the quest for finding your flow. With this book and the introduction of Prasara yoga, we will find a completely new way to think about how we look and perform yoga in the West.

It is with this that I am pleased to introduce Prasara yoga.

Ryan Hurst
Nationally Ranked USA Junior Gymnastics Team Member
Menatoku Police Judo Team (Osaka, Japan)
RMAX Head Coaching Faculty
Real Creative Health Co. CEO

PART ONE

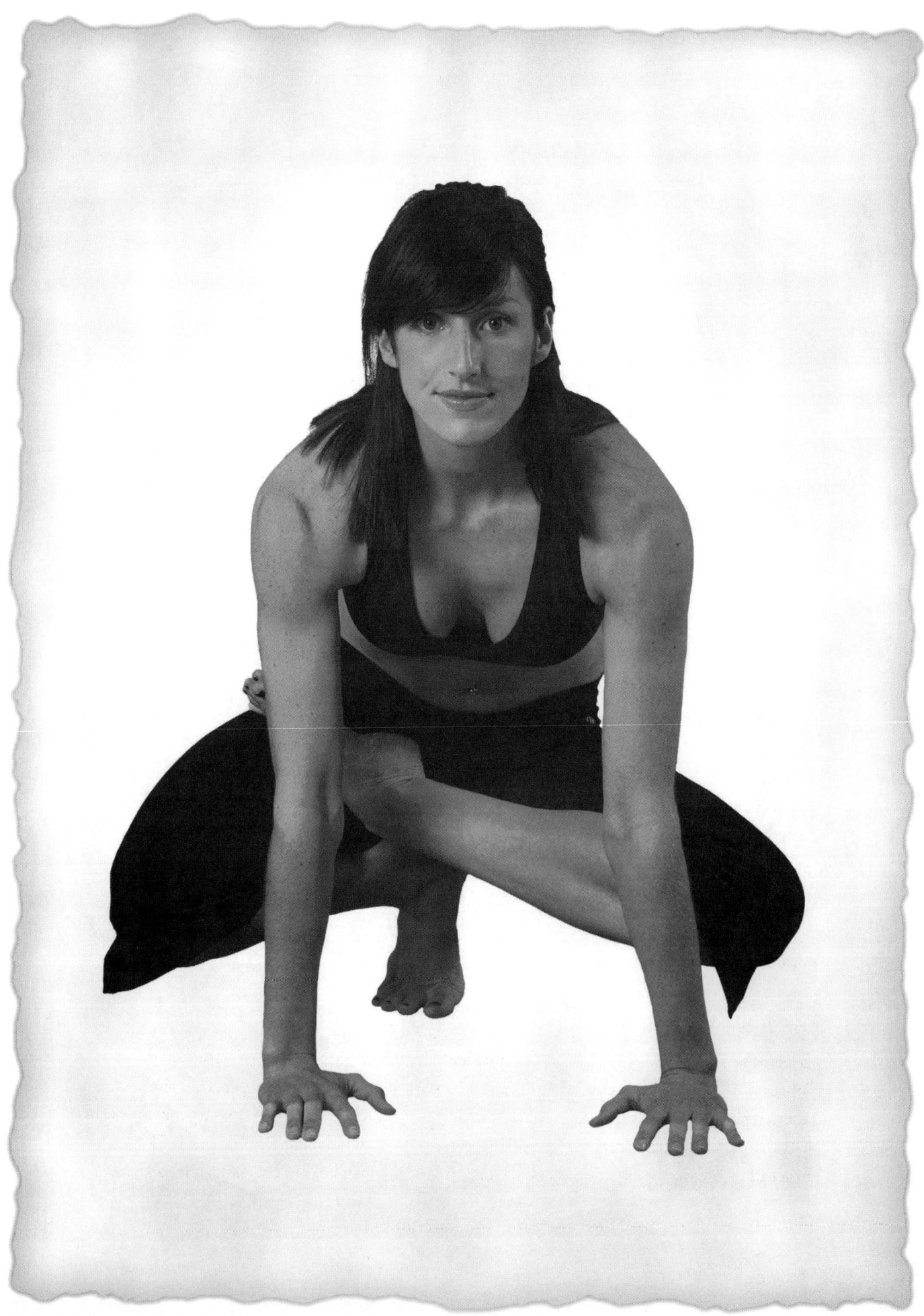

Research Impetus

The author discusses the evolutionary process of yoga through the narrative, dialectic device.

Long ago, in my personal study, I set out to discover if there were core Hatha yoga (the path of physical gymnastics typically understood as "yoga" in the West) principles that governed the movement between asana (postures). In other words, I sought to determine what yoga between the poses was, what sewed their solitary poise together into graceful movement.

A client of mine, a successful yoga school owner, Bri, disclosed some insights on vinyasa as we initially began a conversation about flow in Ashtanga yoga (a particular style of Hatha yoga). Vinyasa is basically a series of yoga postures sequenced together to concentrate on breathing through and between the postures, or asana.

Bri said that although it is mistakenly understood as "movement flows," *vinyasa* actually means a number of yoga postures "linked together in a certain way." She continued on to say that focusing on breathing is the essential ingredient when sequencing asana. The breath must lead the way in the movement from posture to posture. Before a movement, the mind must know exactly where the breath is so that movement and breath are perfectly synchronized.

Since structural alignment is an obvious focus of yoga, when she mentioned this I instantly recognized a universal exercise phenomenon, whether it was Tai Chi Chuan from China, Zdorovye from Russia, or Hatha yoga from India: Flow-state requires the discipline to integrate breath with the structure and movement.

Where's the Mind?

Bri added another important area to consider when performing a vinyasa. The key is "observing thought patterns." A common mistake most people make in practice, she said, is allowing the mind to move ahead of everything else, which it will do as soon as concentration is broken. The mind is in the next posture before the individual has left the prior. The regular practice of breathing techniques, asana, and meditation can help in this area, she explained.

PRASARA YOGA: *Flow Beyond Thought*

Bri continued on that vinyasa is intended to be practiced interwoven with special mantras — poems sculpted around the sequences. The use of the mantras can begin after years of practice of the basic asana, when the body can be calmed through synchronizing breath so that the mind becomes passive throughout the sequences. Bri stated that these mantras have been lost in the modern popularization of yoga.

YOGA THAT ISN'T FIXED

I asked Bri if the postures were removed from the vinyasa, wouldn't it stop the mind from traveling ahead, or rather, wouldn't it stop the mind from abiding in a fixed position. She said of course that would be the goal: to keep in flow.

I then asked if she had ever excluded the perfection of individual postures and experimented particularly with the flow in between. She said that she would need to think about it because what would yoga be without asana?

Bri commented that breathing guides the way between poses. She further stated that movement happens by concentrating on the breathing. I asked her if structural alignment held importance during the movement between asana. She said she would assume so but none of her teachers specifically taught her such.

ZENO'S PARADOX: INFINITE DIGRESSION AND MOVEMENT IMPOSSIBILITY

Bri looked at me, discovering where I had been going with my line of logic. She said, "So you consider yoga vinyasa to be a kinetic chain of an infinite number of asana?" I replied that I considered vinyasa to be a critical step in that direction because before movement can hold flow, it must first have breath synchronously integrated.

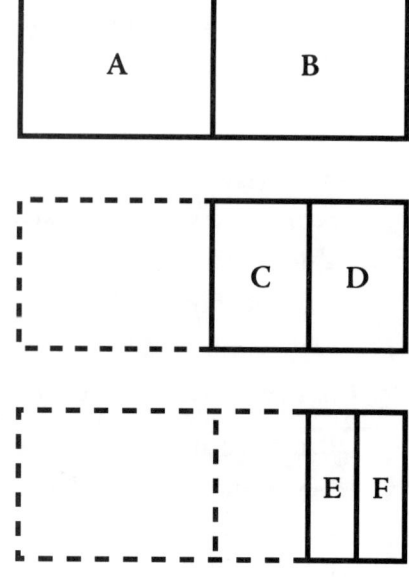

Movement from point B to point A has an infinite number of points in between. In order to travel the distance between the two original points, we must travel half-way, from D to C. And to travel that new distance, we must go half of that (from point F to point E), and half of that, ad infinitum in digression. The paradox is that we will never get to the second point because of the infinite number of places we must be in between to travel from the first point.

PRASARA YOGA: *Flow Beyond Thought*

Bri chuckled at the silliness of such a logic problem because we obviously move all the time and have no problem getting from point A to point B. I told her she had solved one of Zeno's paradoxes by practical sense, but I asked her to explain why it was so. She said that we do not abide at any one of the points in between point A and point B. Rather, we just move through them.

Zeno's paradoxes are a set of paradoxes devised by Zeno of Elea to support Parmenides' doctrine that "all is one" and that contrary to the evidence of our senses, the belief in plurality and change is mistaken, and in particular that motion is nothing but an illusion. Zeno's arguments are perhaps the first examples of a method of proof called *reductio ad absurdum*, also known as proof by contradiction. They are also credited as a source of the dialectic method used by Socrates (and used in the presentation of the author's research impetus).

THE ARROW PARADOX

"You cannot even move. If everything when it occupies an equal space is at rest, and if that which is in locomotion is always occupying such a space at any moment, the flying arrow is therefore motionless." (Aristotle, *Physics*, VI:9, 239b5.)

In the arrow paradox, we imagine an arrow in flight. At every moment in time, the arrow is located at a specific position. If the moment is just a single instant, then the arrow does not have time to move and is at rest during that instant. Now, during the following instants, it then must also be at rest for the same reason. The arrow is always at rest and cannot move; motion is presumed impossible.

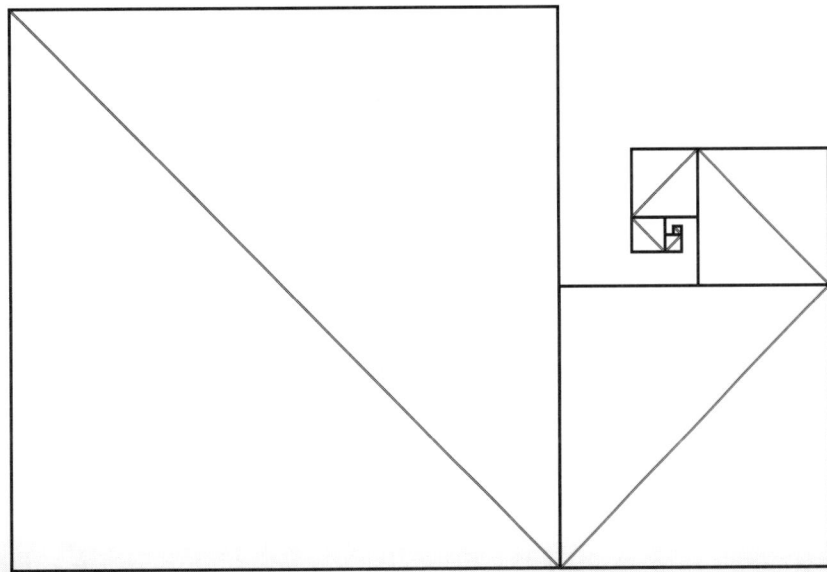

PRASARA YOGA: *Flow Beyond Thought*

NO ABIDING PLACE

"Abide nowhere in particular." (Takuan Soho, *The Unfettered Mind*.)

The solution to Zeno's paradox is that we are never at any point in time, but merely passing through it. I then asked Bri if there were any inherent stopping points in life at all where we would abide (aside from dysfunctional abiding, such as attachments and desires).

She tilted her head, slightly stunned by an apparent shift in the conversation, but then answered, "The only stopping points most people would consider would be birth and death." I hadn't expected such a profound answer. Typically people just answer no. I thanked her. In truth, even birth and death are themselves only points of transition from one energy form to the next.

Continuing onward I stated that if birth is point A and death is point B, then we never abide at any point in time, but rather just move through them over the course of our lifetime. With narrowed eyes, curious where I went with the conversation, Bri answered "Yes." We both conceded that even birth and death are not stopping points but transitional movement in the ultimate cycle of things.

I asked Bri if she would agree then that life is like one's own personalized vinyasa. Her eyebrows lifted, a smile creased across her face, warming her charming little features, and she said, "That's lovely! Yes, of course, that's what life is like! Vinyasa is the micro of the macro where we learn to use breath to move between events."

That led me to my next question: If vinyasa is the micro of the macro, then what is the value of asana?

Bri said that the value is to teach proper structural alignment. However, I was reminded that earlier we had discussed that vinyasa comprised an infinite string of postures in which we are learning to discipline the breath through and between. She replied that the ultimate goal was to remove blockages so that the current of life force that animates us (named *prana* in Sanskrit) could flow unimpeded.

Since movement comprised an infinite number of postures, I asked Bri how the movement between those particular poses had been selected to discipline the breath. She stated, "Only the [founding yogi] would know that answer, I guess."

ONGOING EVOLUTION

Bri wondered about the mental drift from one pose to the next. If asana were excluded, would her students' minds not remain in flow, never abiding? Would this not also coincide with the ultimate goal of yoga, which she defined earlier in the conversation?

PRASARA YOGA: *Flow Beyond Thought*

I suggested to her that like any of the founding yogi she could create her own unique poses upon that infinite line between two points. Once she understood the principles of structure, movement, and breathing, she could even dispense with orthodox poses. Shaking her head back and forth she said, "That's only very advanced yoga. I'm nowhere near that." I asked why if she had such a thorough understanding of structure, breathing, and movement.

Bri looked at me, still flabbergasted, and stuttered, "So you think I should just quit asana?" I asked her if she ever came up with remedial increments on asana that were very challenging to a particular individual. She replied, "I often have to create steps, or *krapa* as they're named in Sanskrit." So she had created variations on asana, which were not orthodoxy.

I also asked Bri if she ever had to modify the steps in between poses in vinyasa so that she or her students could keep the breath in sync with the structure in motion. She replied, "Sure. I must create helpful krapa there as well."

I proposed the idea that if she considered the yogic goal was to decongest life force, then she could target specific issues within her and her students by composing variations of asana if she needed.

Most conventional Westernized yoga practices concentrate on asana. The next evolution beyond building structure (asana) and linking breath (vinyasa) is improvisational flow to explore, locate, and release deeper or more stubborn blockages. This method of yoga, coming after education in asana and vinyasa, is called prasara, which specializes in grace. If asana were the alphabet and vinyasa the grammar, then prasara would be the conversation.

Conventional Westernized yoga does indeed utilize techniques in breathing, posture, and movement to address the individual's daily challenges and exploration. However, a deliberately graduated process of learning the integration of these techniques is not understood or taught: structure through asana, breathing through vinyasa, and flow through prasara.

Reclaiming the Personal Process

I asked Bri if she would be going back to her school to create her own unique flow, to which she stopped and turned around, snickering in shock. She said, "How could I do that? Only the founding yogi can do that."

Knowing that a useful metaphorical interpretation of *yoga* was "yoke" or, in other words, the path to unite with the divine Source, I asked her, "Whose yoga do you practice? Are you following your path or someone else's?"

PRASARA YOGA: *Flow Beyond Thought*

As she pondered the question, I hugged and reminded her that she had already incorporated elements of Pilates, Feldenkrais, Alexander, and Laban into her yoga school. I asked if the founding yogi taught her this, and she chuckled.

I went on to ask her, "What is the difference between those modifications to your path and working within the Hatha yoga structure to create your own unique asana and compose your own unique vinyasa and your own unique flow, or prasara?" She admitted there was none.

Bri let me participate in her next class, to which I had walked with her. She is a superb teacher and helped me target bound areas of tension that my structure had been holding. After the absolutely amazing session, she approached me and said that she saw how to liberate her path from her perceived expectations of long-gone teachers and attachments to self-imposed dogma on how she ought to be teaching.

We are each on our own path. Teachers are critical, but we must remember that their path is not our path. Our way is not their way. We must help others realize that they should not do as their teachers did but seek what they sought. We should take guidance from our teachers and create our own way from their example of how they lived their lives.

Defining Prasara

Prasara Yoga and the Spirit of Patanjali

We have had some idea of the practice of yoga here in America for at least the last hundred years, in Europe for somewhat longer. In the early part of the 20th century, Paramhansa Yogananda introduced the percepts of yoga to a wide Western audience with his Self-Realization Fellowship, including the idea of Hatha yoga.

Hatha yoga is an expression of one of the "eight limbs" (Ashtanga) of yoga as defined by Patanjali in the Sadhana Pada of the Yoga Sutras. The particular limb is Asana, which literally means "to sit" or "a posture." Interestingly, *Hatha* means "force" or "violence," which gives the phrase *Hatha yoga* a possible meaning of "union by force."

Without a doubt, the person who fundamentally defined Hatha yoga in the West was Tirumalai Krishnamacharya, the teacher of such luminaries as B. K. S. Iyengar, T. K. F. Desikachar, and K. Pattabhi Jois. Of the three students, Iyengar could be said to have laid the foundations for today's Hatha yoga with his impeccable attention to the structure of postures.

In the mid-1970s we saw the emergence of a "new" idea within the yoga community with the introduction of K. Pattabhi Jois' Ashtanga Vinyasa yoga.

Vinyasa: The Art of Breath

When K. Pattabhi Jois introduced his yoga to the West he gave us a new concept, that of vinyasa, or "placing in order."

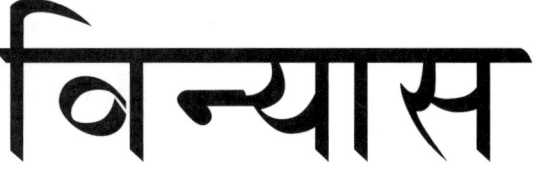

Many people suggest that the Sanskrit word *vinyasa* means "flow"; it does not. The word comes from the root *nyāsa*, which means "putting down or in, placing, fixing, inserting, applying, impressing." The *vi* as a prefix means "division, distinction, distribution, arrangement, order."

Ashtanga Vinyasa gave us the concept that the various asana had a meaningful relationship to each other, and the first, second, and third series of asana developed by Jois reflect this. Not

PRASARA YOGA: *Flow Beyond Thought*

only are the postures arranged in a specific order, but the transitions between each posture are accomplished by integrating breathing techniques with the transitions.

This could be thought of as the "second evolution" of yoga in the West, the idea that the postures of Hatha yoga have a meaningful relationship and that the transitions between them are in some way important.

Prasara: The Art of Movement

A new expression of yoga has recently emerged, one that perhaps adheres more closely to the original scientific foundation of the Yoga Sutras than any other. The creator/rediscover of this yoga method, the author, has named it Prasara yoga.

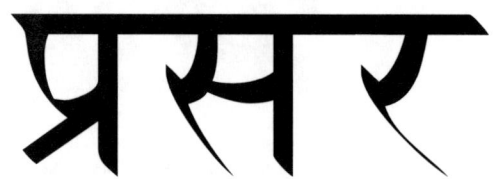

The word *prasara* means "extension, advancing, a free course, a stream." It also carries the meaning of "boldness and courage." Interestingly, when used in the context of music, prasara is a kind of dance.

The word is made from the root *sara*, which means "liquid," "motion," and "going," and the prefix *pra*, which means "forward," "going forth."

Prasara is unique among yoga teachings in that it fully integrates the threefold practice of Kriya yoga and all of the eight limbs of Ashtanga yoga as laid out in the Sadhana Pada of the Yoga Sutras. Furthermore, it is perhaps the only yoga today that explicitly and systematically teaches the eighth limb, Samadhi.

Flow: The Eighth Limb of Yoga

Some experience can be spoken of only through metaphor. This often presents a problem when attempting to transfer knowledge from one culture to another because every culture has its own unique understanding of the symbolism of its metaphor.

There is a state that can be experienced through various means. When we in the West talk about this state we use the metaphoric symbolism of liquid and movement and come up with terms such as *flow*, *flow-state*, and *the zone*.

When Patanjali talked about this state he pulled a different sort of imagery from his cultural milieu and spoke in terms of "union, completion, bringing into harmony, profound attention, and absorption in the present moment" and called the state Samadhi.

PRASARA YOGA: *Flow Beyond Thought*

One of the problems we encounter with most modern yoga teachings is an implicit idea that Samadhi just sort of happens, almost by accident, after long work. The reason for this may be that the specific techniques that develop Samadhi have been lost.

As a matter of fact, even referring to Samadhi as a state may be incorrect from the point of view of the Yoga Sutras. It may be more accurate to say that Samadhi is the practice that produces the state in question.

In his book *Flow-Fighting and the Flow-State Performance Spiral: Peak Performance in Combat Sports*, the author developed the first Western (in the sense of being taught in the native language of the area without reference to outside "loan words"), scientific (in the sense of being based on observation and experimentation, with repeatable results) description of the practice of Samadhi.

This understanding, with the explicit practices that emerge from it, is a foundational pillar of yoga.

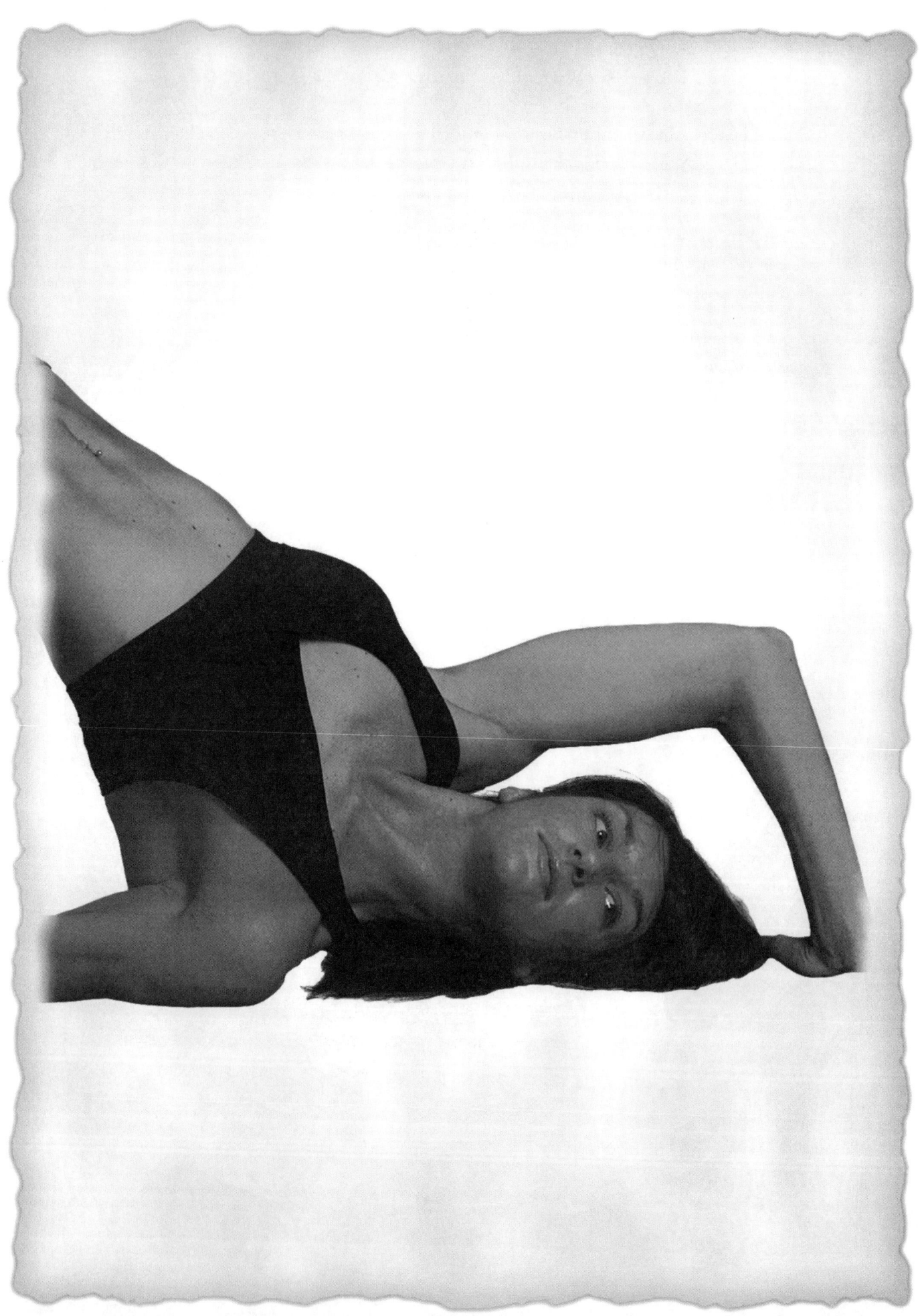

Finding a Balanced Perspective of Hatha Yoga

Often we find ourselves on the fringe in our representation of Hatha yoga — the physical "exercise" approach the West knows as yoga. Commercialized, pop yoga tends to view asana as a series of stretches to increase flexibility. Some better teachers present yoga as a release from chronic tension, the "yin" aspect that has become so popular. But why has this singular aspect of yoga gained such strong representation?

Presumably, the answer lies in what a particular society needs in general. Yoga has a balancing effect not only on the individual but on the collective group. With the domination of the bodybuilding, powerlifting, and cross-training belief systems, these overly masculine, imbalanced systems create a social need for their corollary opposite pole: Yin yoga. Chronic tension, whether or not from beliefs like in conventional so-called fitness, begs the attraction of the yielding, softer feminine.

Yin yoga is more than mere exercise selection; it is a protocol. In yoga classes, you hear this as the need to "surrender" — to relax, melt, release, and unlock. But too much surrender is a danger, just like joints too loose are a danger.

There must be a balance of strength and surrender in any structure, in any relationship. Like a tensegrity structure, the human form comprises strong, stable compressive struts pushing out within the sea of continuous tension pulling in to create "zero" — the antigravitational efficiency of the (unimpeded) human gait.

Too much surrender is like loosening the high-tension wires holding up the mast of a sailboat. When a strong wind comes and suddenly fills the sails, the mast will snap. The hypermobile, overly flexible joints of some proponents in Western commercialized yoga are no better than the distorted tissues of a contortionist. That approach is just unsafe and unhealthy.

Yoga itself means "to unite." Interestingly, *Hatha* means "force" or "violence," which gives the phrase *Hatha yoga* a possible meaning of "union by force."

PRASARA YOGA: *Flow Beyond Thought*

If we were to remove the social demands, which have attracted only one aspect of yoga to the West, how would yoga appear? If commercialized yoga were not a compensation for the chronic tension of bodybuilding, powerlifting, and cross-training, how would it appear as a path unto itself?

It would be a balancing act of moving between strength and surrender, heading toward that optimal relationship of zeroing out excess, of the "middle road" that Buddhists talk about.

Yoga should be as much about the act of surrender as it is a battle against our ego's tyranny over our health. Yoga isn't usually held in this light in the West, and instead is held to be that flaccid, doe-eyed expression that most people mistake for bliss. But even if we look to yoga's country of origin, in the Bhagavad Gita we see imperatives uttered by Krishna, an incarnation of God, to Arjuna before going into battle:

> "Fix your mind on the eternal self, be without any thought of mine, put away your agitation, and fight." (Lesson 3, verses 30–32.)

> "At all times remember me, and fight." (Lesson 8, verses 1–8.)

From Patanjali's Yoga Sutras, we find the following (translations by Mushtaq Ali Al-Ansari, Ph.D.):

- **rupa-lavaya-bala-vajra-samhanantvani kaya-sampat:** Symmetry of form, beauty of color, strength, and the compactness of the diamond constitute bodily perfection.

- **mrdu-madhya-adhimatratvat tato'pi visesah:** Because of the mild, the medium, and the transcendent nature of the methods adopted, there is a distinction to be made among those who practice yoga.

- **tato dvandva-anabhighatah:** The fruit of right poise is the strength to resist the shocks of infatuation or sorrow. When this condition has been attained, the yogi feels no assaults from the pairs of opposites.

There's nothing namby-pamby milquetoast about that guidance. There is a very clear notion of action, of strength, of balancing the masculine and feminine, of yang with the yin.

When practicing your yoga, remember that you are a unique relationship of selective tension, moving in a field of various pulls and pushes. Flow-state, known as the eighth limb of yoga, or Samadhi, is the balance of zeroing out excess — not too much tension, not too much relaxation, not too much strength, not too much surrender. It's a never-ending path of compensating for swinging too far to one side here, too far to the other side there.

PRASARA YOGA: *Flow Beyond Thought*

When we stop trying to do yoga a certain way, when we cease thinking yoga is a "thing" unto itself and realize that it is another tool for balance in our lives, we stop *doing* yoga altogether and start *being* yoga.

We will continue our discussion by redefining the three evolutions of personal practice of yoga — asana, vinyasa, and prasara — within this new, balanced perspective.

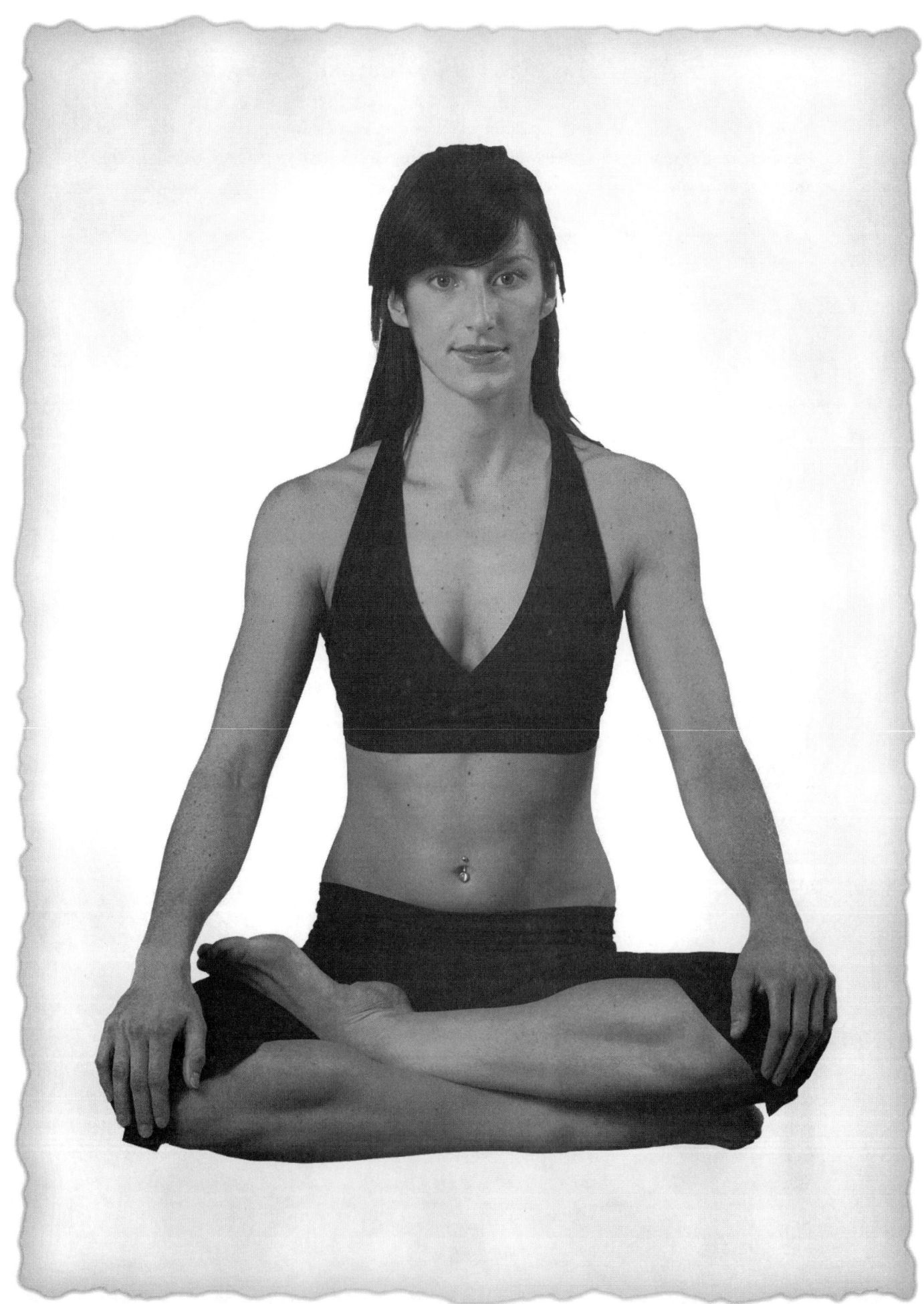

Defining Asana in Exercise Physiology

Commercialized, pop yoga tends to view asana as a series of stretches to increase flexibility. The author intends in this section to redefine the physiological event of an asana, or structure, and how it relates to enabling or disinhibiting flow in vinyasa and, eventually, prasara.

Athletes are told incessantly to stretch out our muscles before and after exercising. However, when most people say "stretch" they mean to take a muscle and force it to lengthen until it changes shape and stays longer. This is analogous to taking a rubber band, lengthening it, tacking it down, and, over time, observing how the rubber band loses its elasticity and adopts the new length.

The danger is that our joints need this elasticity in order to protect themselves, to keep everything packed tightly. Dancers, gymnasts, and contortionists — arguably the most flexible people in the world — suffer debilitating injuries in later life due to permanent changes in tissue length. The lax, loose connective tissue is not able to keep them from hypermobile injuries.

Much of commercialized, pop yoga approaches asana as stretches. This is a basic misunderstanding of Hatha yoga asana based upon the filter of traditional static stretching to deform the plastic region of connective tissue. However, dynamic and static mobility isn't about stretching in the above sense. Asana are dynamic postures that apply the concept of reciprocal inhibition: Flexion of one causes a release of its twin. (Dr. Mel Siff, *Supertraining*.) For instance, in Standing Half-Moon Pose, the goal is not to stretch the hamstrings but to pull the heels to the chest as hard as possible; thereby, the hamstrings cannot maintain their tension.

Yoga is a balance of strength and surrender, not stretching (as in the conventional usage of the term). Flexibility is a measure of the increased range of motion due to an improved strength/surrender ratio. We never use flexibility in real life; it's a measure alone. It's analogous to using the bench press as a measure of one's ability to function in daily life — an arbitrary measurement.

PRASARA YOGA: *Flow Beyond Thought*

Dynamic range of motion, or the ability to move through, about, and around all other flexibility measurements for a specific joint(s), is much more applicable to daily life. Dynamic mobility is not a measurement (one cannot measure the range infinity in basic mathematics); it's reality.

To understand this paradigm shift from commercialized, pop yoga as a form of static stretching, the author now presents a deeper physiological appreciation of the event of yoga asana.

Soviet scientist and physician Alexander Bogomoletz said wisely, "Man is as old as his connective tissues." The corollary to this statement is expressed in the title to Editha Hearn's 1967 book *You Are as Young as Your Spine*. Basically, if we rely on tissue elasticity for flexibility, we'll lose it. We must master the regulation of selective tension through asana in order to gain dynamic strength to move from vinyasa to prasara.

Tendons do not have to be maximally stretched to be torn. Tears are the result of a special combination of sudden stretch and muscular contraction.

Everyone has slipped on ice at one point in their lives. If we slip on the ice, our body is thrown off balance. It reflexively attempts to restabilize the breach of stance integrity. The tissue we stretch when we slip, say the hamstring or groin, will contract to the original position. Voila! We experience a tear: a stretch from one side and a simultaneous contraction on the other. This involuntary event is called the stretch reflex: A muscle that is stretched by an external force too far or too fast will contract to oppose the stretch.

Before beginning dynamic strengthening exercises to develop plasticity, we must learn to regulate the muscular tension. This is not as difficult as it sounds, but it requires a paradigm shift from conventional methods.

Debunking the Stretching Myth

Stretching is not considered a particularly high-premium healthy characteristic. Stretching has been a buzz word, and rarely has anyone been given the opportunity to question whether this is a virtue for health and longevity by increasing flexibility.

We have seen a significant deterioration of connective tissue strength and pervasive injuries in every sport and at every age through the dangerous stretching practices of the conventional fitness industry. There are important myths to overcome. Some of these myths are listed here and then debunked:

- Flexibility is the primary characteristic of health and sportive/combative performance. The more flexible, the better.

PRASARA YOGA: *Flow Beyond Thought*

- Flexibility is a form of injury prevention.
- Injury results from insufficient warm-up to increase flexibility.
- Injury happens when tissue is stretched maximally.
- Static stretching is safe and productive; dynamic stretching (mobility training and ballistic motion) is unsafe and unproductive.
- Daily stretching is mandatory for flexibility maintenance.
- Flexibility requires many years and is the first characteristic lost.
- (The most terrible) Flexibility is gained through elongating the tissues (deformation).

FLEXIBILITY VERSUS ELASTICITY

Flexibility is a measurable range of motion in one specific direction. To increase the flexibility of a tissue, we must apply a force pulling the tissue in an isolated range of motion until the stress causes a permanent deformation of the tissue, where it will not return to its original state.

However, over years and a lifetime, we cause micro trauma to our tissue from activity. The tissue heals, but only after scar tissue has formed. In healing, the scar tissue mends the wound together by pulling and shortening the tissue.

Many people, in conventional understanding of physical culture, have made the assumption that stretching after activity can prevent the muscle from healing at a shorter length. However, should the stretching manage to prevent shortening (which is debatable), the connective tissues will stiffen regardless. Tendons and ligaments are composed of collagen (lending tensile strength) and elastin (lending elasticity, obviously). As we age, our tissues endure an irreversible process of increasing collagen and decreasing elastin.

Elasticity is a material's ability to return to its original state following deformation after removal of the deforming load. To increase the elasticity of a tissue, we must apply a load to the tissue in a range of motion, then remove the load, after the initial stiffness ceases (discomfort, not pain) and before the tissue is permanently deformed so that the tissue returns to its original state. This stress increases the capacity for storage of elastic energy.

STORED ELASTIC ENERGY AND VISCOSITY

The ability to generate stored elastic energy (SEE) is proportionate to the tensile strength of the tissue. Tensile strength is the maximum stress that a material can withstand before it breaks. The ductility (how malleable a substance is) decreases as a material reaches its tensile strength failure; conversely, the amount of SEE increases as a material reaches its tensile strength failure.

This is the concept of viscosity: the property of an object that demonstrates that a body at rest tends to stay at rest unless acted upon by an outside force. Many tissues of the human body exhibit constricting, congealing, and thickening characteristics when not exposed to outside forces. The viscosity of a tissue is its resistance to the force: The greater the viscosity, the greater the force and time required to cause deformation.

To understand this concept, we pull a rubber band in two opposite directions. The more that we pull, the harder it is to pull. For example, if we pull the rubber band one inch, it gains 5 units of SEE; if we pull one more inch, it produces 10 additional units of SEE (15 total); if we pull one final inch, it results in 20 more units of SEE (35 total). The increase is exponential. The more we pull the rubber band, the farther it will fly when we release one side.

Tissues adapt to both the intensity and the duration of the stress placed upon them. So two things can occur. In the rubber band example, too much stress can cause the rubber band to snap, or the rubber band can begin to deform permanently.

The Stretch Reflex

If the tensile strength of the rubber band is 50 units and we pull the rubber band one final inch (which should produce 40 more units of SEE, for a total of 75), the tensile strength of the rubber band has been exceeded. Failure has resulted, and it snaps in two. High degrees of flexibility outside of the natural range of motion of the joint make snapping much more likely.

Some teachers have used this knowledge to make a leap in logic that injuries occur when a muscle is stretched beyond its limit. Therefore, one ought to prevent injuries by elongating the muscles of the connective tissues.

This assumption is a physiological falsehood. Tears do not happen because tissues have been maximally stretched (as the stretching pundits would have us believe) but due to the special combination of sudden stretch and contraction called the stretch reflex.

The stretch reflex is where the tissue that is stretched by an external force too far or too fast will contract to oppose the stretch. When a stretch from one side happens simultaneous to a contraction on the other, we have a tear. We have seen this frequently in the dance and fitness industry, and unfortunately as a result of the recent craze in the pollution of the yoga discipline (where commercialized, pop yoga represents itself as static stretching).

PRASARA YOGA: *Flow Beyond Thought*

Viscoelasticity: Flexibility Is Speed Specific

The belief exists that if we maintain a certain pull length on the rubber band for an extended time (say at 35 units), the rubber band will begin to deform permanently, and as a result lose SEE as it loses its degree of elasticity. This region of training is known as viscoelasticity: having a combination of viscosity and elasticity.

Viscoelastic materials have time-dependent mechanical properties, being sensitive to the duration of the force application. Such materials will continue to deform over a finite length of time, even if the load remains constant, until a state of equilibrium is reached (also known as the "creep effect").

High temperatures increase the rate of creep and low temperatures decrease it. For the most effective use of this property, the material to be deformed should be warmed and then have a sufficient load applied over a long period of time. Different tissues respond differently to various rates of loading. When loaded rapidly, they exhibit greater resistance to deformation than if they are loaded slowly.

This is why dynamic flexibility cannot be gained through static stretches. Flexibility is speed specific. The stretch reflex engages whenever a muscle is stretched suddenly or dramatically, or both. This mechanism is controlled by the muscle spindles, which are two special receptors that activate the stretch reflex. One of these is sensitive to stretch magnitude and the other is sensitive to speed and magnitude. The prevalent static stretch may or may not reset the first receptor, but it is completely ineffective for the latter. As a result, flexibility is speed specific.

Health Risks of Static Stretching

The practice of increasing flexibility through static stretching in the fitness industry is standard. This is a serious health danger. As we have seen, with age the collagen/elastin ratio changes in favor of collagen. So as we grow older, with the decreased integrity of the tissue elasticity, the connective tissue is more likely to snap.

In our youth, dropping into a straddle split seemed like a desirable ability, but it has nothing to do with health, and even less to do with longevity. As we grow older, we see that it is not how far in a particular direction we can move that is important but how strong our tissues are, how quickly they resolve deviations in movement and afford us mobile security.

As a result, the first training emphasis is to be flexible in motion (what the author terms "real-world flexibility"). We must coordinate range of mobility, and eventually at our activity's velocity.

PRASARA YOGA: *Flow Beyond Thought*

Short-Range Stiffness

Most people tend to feel better after they've gone through a stretching routine. They are likely to feel loose and more relaxed. This is healthy but should be properly understood. Physiologically, when inactive we experience short-range stiffness (SRS), which is a mechanical property of the muscle tissue whereby the stiffness is high for the first few millimeters of the stretch. After surpassing this initial short resistance, there is a substantial reduction in the stiffness of the tissue. This is a temporary physiological phenomenon, not a permanent one.

We should concentrate on overcoming the SRS, but not proceed to deformation of the tissue. Static stretching is not a means for permanently remaining flexible. Attempting to alter the mechanical properties of our tissues may work when we are children, but it does not work in developed adults. The goal of allowing the organism to be permanently flexible is achieved through the regulation of muscular tension — governing the stretch reflex.

Plasticity Changes

Plasticity is at the far end of the spectrum from elasticity. It is the quality of a connective tissue, such as a ligament or tendon, when subjected to ballistic, prolonged, or sudden forces exceeding the elastic limits of the tissue. The tissue does not return to its original state after the deforming load is removed. The anatomical plastic region (APR) of connective tissue is found between 6% and 10% of the ligament's or tendon's resting length, and is at the very wall of failure (to the maximum tissue tensile strength).

From plasticity, we learn that some tissues are less injury prone when stressed rapidly. For instance, ligaments are composed of wavy collagen fibers. Uncoiled, the fibers become taught and susceptible to injury. If taken into the APR, a ligament tears. Whereas slow loading causes uncoiling through taking the slack out of the fibers, quick loading does not allow sufficient time for a ligament to enter the APR.

The properties of cartilage make it equally less injury prone when quickly loaded. Cartilage decreases the stress in a joint by decreasing the friction coefficient between bones and through distributing load over the surface of the joint complex. Cartilage is composed of 20–40% collagen and 60–80% water. With predictability, cartilage behaves with the properties of water in a sponge. When it is compressed it decreases the protection between bones. However, with rapid loading the fluid does not have sufficient time to be squeezed out and the shock absorption is maximal.

Discomfort is productive; pain is unproductive. This statement is completely subjective, and there must be a dialogue/feedback between our teacher and ourselves, or at the very least between our journal or weblog and ourselves.

PRASARA YOGA: *Flow Beyond Thought*

We do not stretch in isolation for its own sake. We do not stretch in isolation (since isolation is the most virulent myth) to induce permanent deformation of the tissue to increase flexibility. To begin increasing the plasticity of the body, we stretch locally until the short-range stiffness is removed. This is a very short and insignificant aspect of preparation. Then we move to engage the organism through a complete range of motion.

There are simple biomechanics involving one joint matrix (such as large arm circles through the 135-degree range of motion), and there are complex ranges of motion comprising multijoint matrixes, which must be modeled and then experienced kinesthetically. All of this information leads to the conclusion that the primary characteristic of maximal flexibility is in the regulation of the stretch reflex through sensitivity to muscular tension and the cultivation of plasticity and viscoelasticity of tissues through yoga.

MOBILITY — THE ANTIAGING AGENT

Mobility practice is more important for not only athletic performance but also antiaging. Dynamic mobility is most often used for an energetic supercharge, as well as a warm-up for more strenuous activities. Another important use for mobility practice is as an active recovery session or cycle when we don't want to train strenuously.

Flexibility, on the other hand, means the elasticity of the tissues. With conventional flexibility training we use static stretching (with the help of gravity, a partner or object leveraged to increase length).

Mobility means movement (not position) into the extreme range of motion of each joint through voluntary muscular control.

Unlike what we would find in flexibility training, in mobility practice we don't try to hold an extreme position. We pass through it slowly and smoothly without forcing the tissues to deform, but rather by allowing the muscles to relax voluntarily.

If one insists on flexibility training, then the author suggests an active contraction release type of stretching known as Proprioceptive Neuromuscular Facilitation (PNF). Although very rigorous, PNF will improve strength. However, because it is so demanding, perform this type of training only at the end of the day, after all other activities conclude.

STATIC STRETCHING VERSUS ASANA

Static stretching, asana, vinyasa, and prasara involve very different agendas. The people who find the most difficulty learning yoga, for instance, are usually the most flexible. The common Western misunderstanding is that yoga is "just stretching," when in reality it is the opposite;

stretching moves against the tension to deform the tissues, whereas asana breathe into the tension to allow it to relax while simultaneously providing stabilizing strengthening.

Asana are a means of surrendering tension through breathing and focus to augment mobility practice. As such, asana can be used when encountering a restricted range of motion in vinyasa or prasara practice. We can select or create an asana to release the tension binding the flow.

We must cultivate an eye for assessing and targeting tension chains prohibiting pain-free, powerful movement. As a result, we can use our intuition to select asana to target prohibitive tension. We can do this by moving into the asana with practice, consistency, and diligence. When we do, we'll be able to release layers of deeper and deeper tension at critical points in our mobility, thus giving us the ability to strengthen even greater mobility, and make mobile even greater strength. Prasara, vinyasa, and asana are three very important and mutually beneficial tools to this end.

Balance and Proprioception

From physical therapy to the hottest glamour gym, fitness enthusiasts everywhere are jumping on the wobbling, jostling, and teetering balance training bandwagon.

From a proprioceptive perspective (i.e., from the perspective of sensory receptors, chiefly in muscles, tendons, and joints responding to stimuli arising from the body), learning balance work is highly specific because the nervous system learns it not in general but relative to the learning of specific skills.

We are able to learn new balance skills more rapidly when the skills we are learning are complex. Some teachers too often wrongly assume, however, that the more rapid acquisition of these new skills is due to a general physical development of the kinesthetic sense rather than an improvement in our ability to focus and concentrate as we learn each new skill.

The mechanical ear of proprioception is mechanoreception (reception that responds to mechanical stimuli such as tension and pressure). One of the three aspects of mechanoreception is movement — or kinesthetic sense. The other two aspects are position sense and force/tension sense. It is important to remember that movement (kinesthetic sense), position sense, and force/tension sense are, in fact, sense aspects of mechanoreception rather than attributes. And they are senses that a person is born with, just as one is born with the senses of sight, hearing, and taste.

Proprioception, then, is not something athletes develop like strength or endurance, but, rather, it is a "sixth" sense athletes have that is critical and that should not be overlooked or ignored.

PRASARA YOGA: *Flow Beyond Thought*

Regarding the recent pop balance culture, unless one intends to compete on a pneumatic wobble surface, or on a playing field on rollers, balance training will transfer more rapidly if it is approached from the top down rather than from the bottom up. Top-down balance training actively perturbs the structural alignment to illicit the body's natural falling defense — the righting reflex.

This righting reflex is hard-wired into the human system, so we cannot alter it. However, skills to coordinate reactions subsequent to the righting reflex can be learned. And we can learn to coordinate our actions so that our center of mass remains aligned with our center of gravity, even when actively facing resistance.

If we lift a leg off the ground and have a friend push us, as our center of mass displaces off of our aligned center of balance, our leg instantly comes down to protect us from the fall. We can, of course, interfere with this by allowing our hands to break our fall. Regardless, righting ourselves so that we do not fall becomes imperative in our mind, overriding all other thoughts. Our mind is rightly concerned with our situation, and designed to be so. It is a matter of survival.

In the yoga flows, there are numerous falling and rolling skills one can learn for engaging the ground. These skills demand extensive conditioning to wire our system. Likewise, in developing balancing skills, this wiring is not balancing that we learn. Rather, it's improving our coordination through learning how to perform various stunts on equipment.

The Dysfunction of Mirrors

This section of the book addresses an educational dictum shared by all Bikram yoga instructors, as it is a technical requirement in the asana sequence — that we must stare into a mirror ahead of us.

Bikram may have had a particular intent in mind: expedient success in the particular pose. And by staring into the mirror, we tap into the trinity of balancing mechanisms in our body:

- **Proprioceptive:** Proprioception involves the sense organs throughout our soft tissue, which instantly inform us of changes in movement, force/tension, and position. Proprioception is the fastest and the most efficient balancing mechanism because it is most directly plugged into our nervous system. However, as we know, it is our proprioception that suffers when we become injured, anxious, or traumatized, leading to a host of compensations (inappropriate tension chains and density) that in turn create the downward spiral of the degeneration of our physical vibrancy.

PRASARA YOGA: *Flow Beyond Thought*

- **Visual:** Our sight is the next fastest and the next most efficient mechanism in our balance, though we tend to rely upon it most heavily. In particular, Bikram in standing postures relies more heavily upon the visual than proprioception through the mirror-staring requirement. This requirement relies upon a particular physiological reflex called the Ocular-Gyro-Cephalic (OGC) reflex, which creates tension chains that reflexively cause the body to orient toward whatever the eyes seek. Alexander Technique names this righting reflex "Primary Control."

  This dependence on vision for balance becomes an issue when we are injured and age. If we do not rewire proprioception, and as we age our sight begins to falter, we are in great danger. By relying upon the OGC reflex, Bikram does not rewire any proprioceptive errors in the system.

  This is why in the prasara forest flow we begin by looking four feet in front of us on the ground, tethering ourselves to the ground. Then, as soon as we relax into the movement, we practice with our eyes closed. In this way we tap into correcting any aberrant issues in our proprioceptive clarity of balance.

- **Vestibular:** There is fluid in the semicircular canals within each of the ears. As we move, this fluid sloshes around. If we're not acclimated to a particular pattern of movement, then we may feel dizzy. Our brain strives to make sense of this novel information, and strikes to integrate it with the stimulus and processing from both our visual and proprioceptor systems. Although some less informed individuals will claim that this is not a factor in this type of balance because it is the slowest mechanism, it is indeed a contributing factor in grace (moving balance).

  Here again there is a problem with the nonmoving pose holding in Bikram yoga compared with the Four-Corner Balance Drill (FCBD). When a pose is held, there is very little movement to stimulate and challenge the vestibular system; whereas in FCBD, there is constant movement and repositioning of the head, causing continual shifts in the inner-ear fluid. Without movement, balance is not developed to its full extent to include vestibular development.

  Bikram yoga's standing postures requiring mirror staring for balance overemphasize our already eye-dominant balance. People will have quick success in achieving the poses. However, it is only an external achievement, and will remain only external.

  To develop the entire organism, to restore true grace that was stolen by trauma, fear, anxiety, or even merely unanswered specialization, which comes from not changing our normal routine throughout the day, we must challenge all

PRASARA YOGA: *Flow Beyond Thought*

three mechanisms: proprioceptive, visual, and vestibular. To do that, we must remove the dominant, the visual, so that the others may catch up in their lagging development. This is why the FCBD is designed in the manner it is: constant movement, eyes close to the ground and eventually closed, head always repositioning.

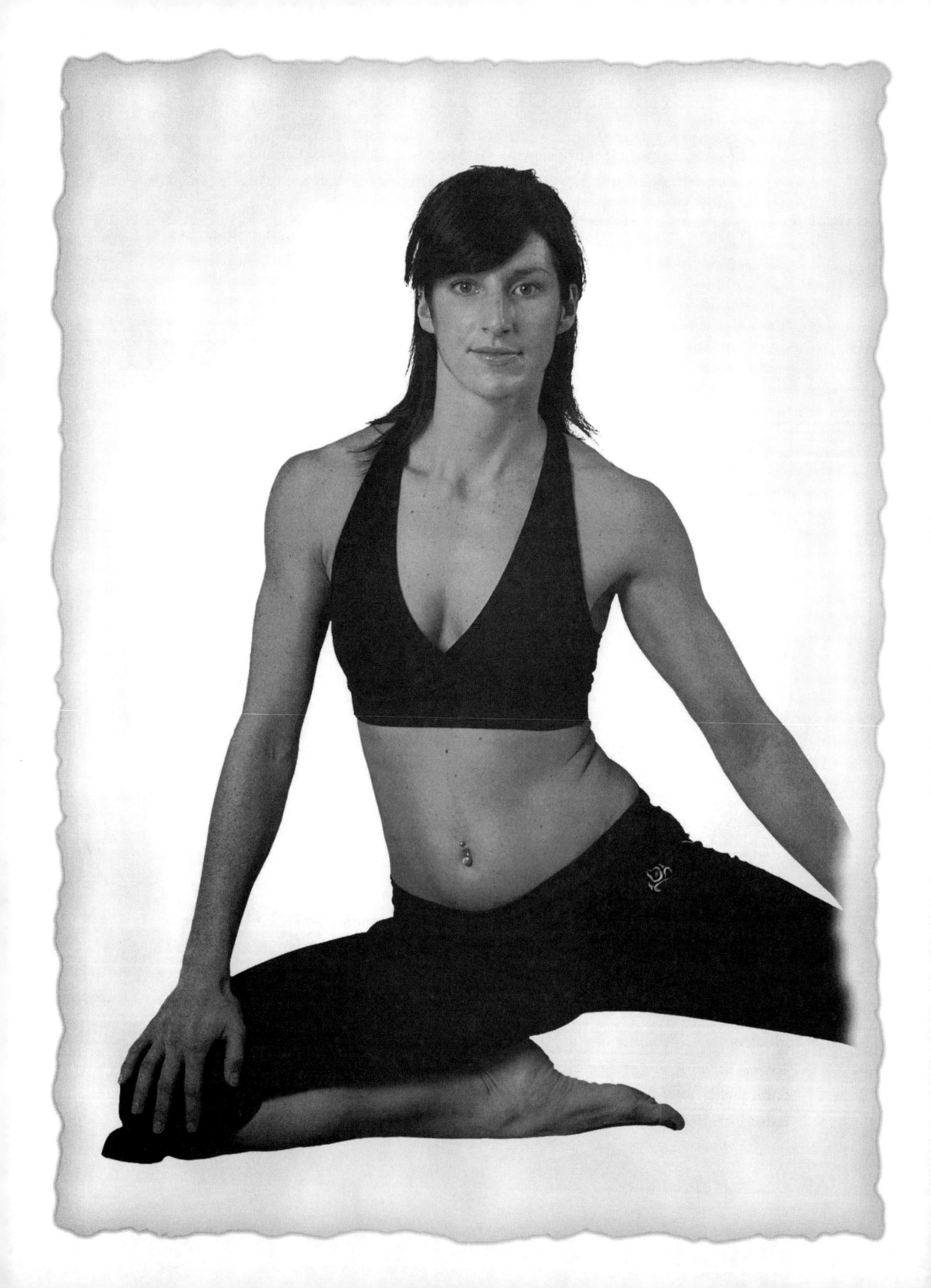

Defining Body Flow in Exercise Physiology

"I am skeptical of science's presumption of objectivity and definitiveness. I have a difficult time seeing scientific results, especially in neurobiology, as anything but provisional approximations, to be enjoyed for a while and discarded as soon as better accounts become available." (Antonio Damasio, *Descartes' Error*.)

This author defines *body flow* as the ability to be fully present during the act of physical existence — a state of unity in which psychological, emotional, and physical energies lack distinction. The author presents that body flow holds the key to better health and well-being through this integrated presence.

Many people discuss how to gain flow in life, but the very investigation taints the exploration. They ask, How do I gain flow? However, it is this very inquiry that arrests the development of those who seek improvement through the physical path.

Body flow is not something to be gained. This is the reason most people do not know how to flow. Body flow is not something we do but something we must get out of the way of. We must get out of the way of our own genius, talent, and abundance — which are our birthright. Body flow is not something to be acquired, but rather something that we will learn to avoid interrupting. A much more appropriate question to ask is, What prevents us from having body flow?

Many people perceive flow as the absence of errors, the condition of never experiencing surprise and shock, never fearing challenge. This is why most lack physical mastery, why they lack grace and poise. They associate "doing their best" with perfection. This creates fear of making mistakes by creating false expectations of performance.

However, it is precisely the experience of failure that opens the gateway to flow. The failures are just scenery along this path. Winston Churchill said, "Success is going from failure to failure without losing enthusiasm." Successful people systematically unhinge themselves from failed expectations. They move from one attachment to the next without being distracted by the appearance of failure. Flow isn't something we can seek, but rather it is the process we unlock by letting go of attachments, by freeing ourselves from expectations.

Dance annotator Rudolf Laban (1879–1958), a pioneer in movement analysis, coined the term *bound flow* as "the stopping point in action." Laban had invented a method that could be used for all observable motion. His book *Labanotation* is used extensively in dance and choreography.

Body flow was one of Laban's critical four elements of analysis, which defined movement as a singular impulse to move restricted to various degrees, or bound, depending upon its function. He felt that the more bound, the more laborious the motion. Less bound, or freer-flowing, movement he associated with emotional expression and creative impulse. When movement is most bound, no visible movement can be seen; whereas when movement is least bound, grace erupts.

So we can define success as the enthusiastic movement from failure to failure without attachment or expectation — without binding flow. We must ask ourselves, What is my current degree of success? How long does it take us to recover from being surprised, shocked, disappointed, frustrated, angered, or dismayed or from any other emotional or mental distraction? How quickly can we regain our composure and enthusiasm and stop resisting the flow of life?

We must challenge or change the training habits and personal beliefs that contribute to our stress and dysfunction — to the blockage of our flow. What is it that we put in our own way? What hurdles do we create for ourselves?

Masterful people perceive making mistakes as a positive influence on performance. They perceive the unexpected as opportunity meeting preparation.

The key to body flow, therefore, rests with deliberate exposure to making mistakes and to unexpected events combined with the proper training protocol, emotional control, and mental attitude. Body flow requires the removal of fear of making mistakes and fear of the unexpected. Our ability to take risks allows us to enter greatness and uncover our personal mastery.

Face challenge by risking mistakes and welcoming unexpected events. We must deliberately engage the areas that we fear. We increase our confidence not by refinement in areas where we are comfortable but by facing the areas where we fear mistakes and the unknown. Our fears inhibit our performance and block our flow.

Flow never attaches anywhere. It never abides. It constantly moves. We must focus on this state of detachment in order to address constantly changing variables. We must seek movement freedom to keep our movement from binding. In reality, stillness can be gained only

PRASARA YOGA: *Flow Beyond Thought*

through continual motion because attempting to stop motion requires force. We always move, even when we try to force ourselves to be still.

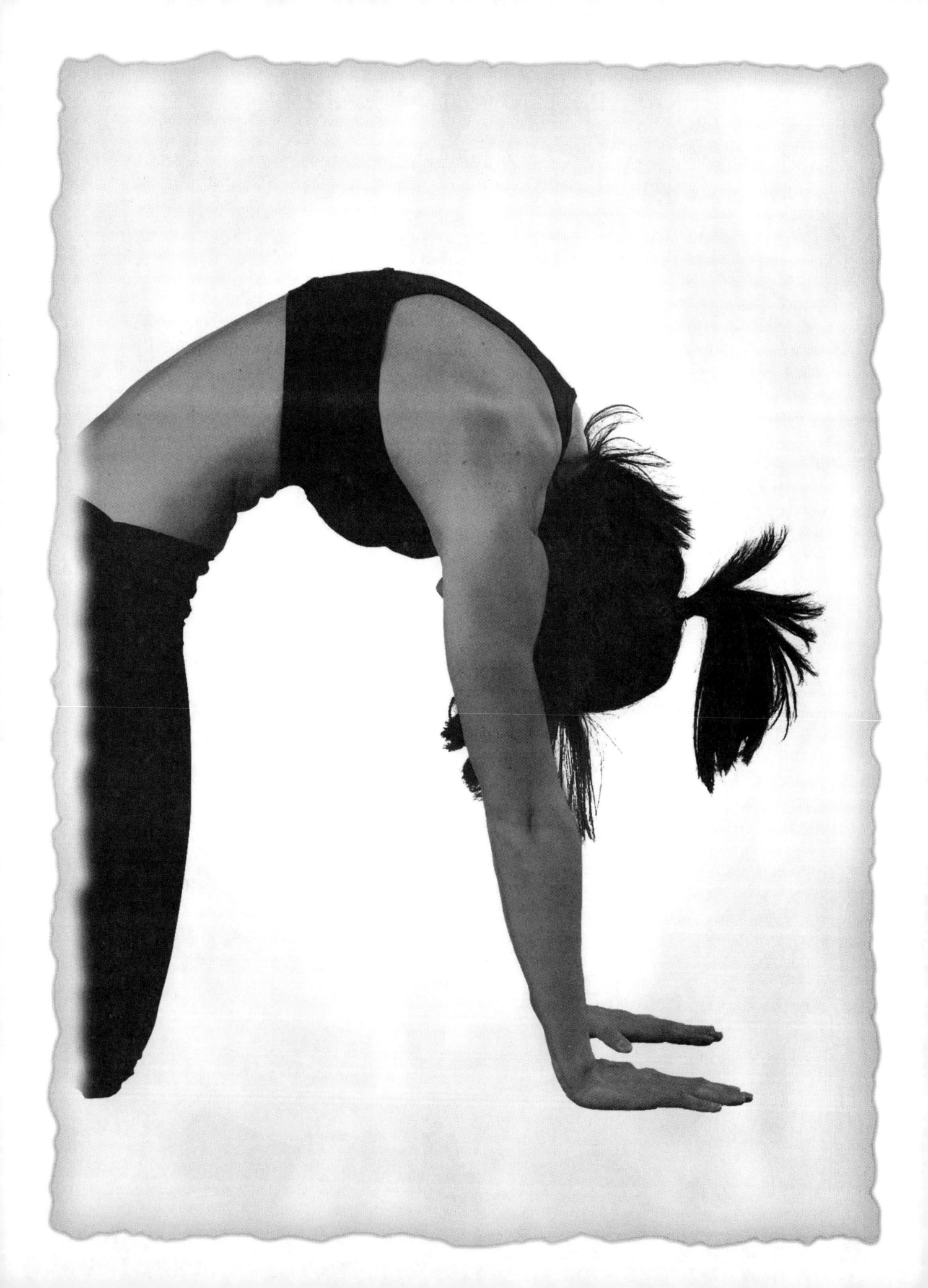

The Progressive Degrees of Body Flow

Refine the integration of breathing, movement, and structure to produce endless improvement in quality of life. Most fitness programs focus on enhancing performance and decreasing injury by focusing upon general calisthenics: squats, push-ups, sit-ups, pull-ups, and so on. These exercises may enhance sport performance but execute essentially in a one-dimensional plane, which can be understood as "linear strength." Linear strength transfers to athletes' hitting harder, running faster, and jumping higher. However, during practice or competition, every sport, and, more important, life in general, demands fluid movement in three planes.

Three Planes of Movement

- **Coronal plane:** The coronal plane divides the body into front and rear sections.

- **Sagittal plane:** The sagittal plane divides the body into right and left sections.

- **Axial, or transverse plane:** The transverse plane divides the body into upper and lower sections.

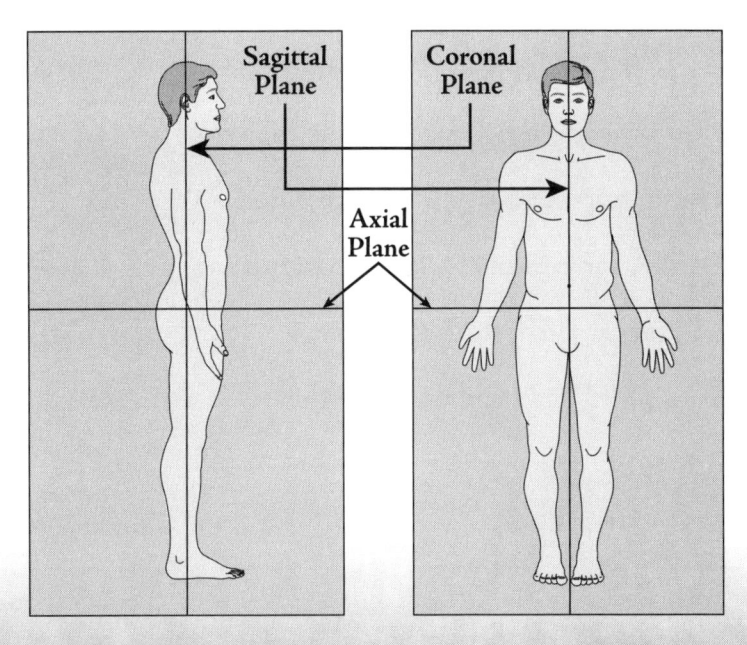

PRASARA YOGA: *Flow Beyond Thought*

Three Axes of Rotation

- **Medial axis:** The medial axis runs horizontally from back to front (e.g., cartwheels and turntables).

- **Longitudinal axis:** The longitudinal axis extends vertically from head to toe (e.g., twisting our torso as in a pirouette).

- **Transverse axis:** The transverse axis runs horizontally across our body from one side of the waist to the other (e.g., somersaults and flips).

Triplanar movements develop rotary and angular/diagonal strength to assist the prime movers. More important, prime movers can act with rotary and angular/diagonal strength, though most people fail to develop this capacity!

Developing multiplanar strength of the prime movers increases stability, enhances injury prevention, multiplies force production abilities, and, most important, stimulates the neuromuscular patterns required of athletes. Prasara yoga, by its movement through the six mechanical degrees of freedom, targets the rotary and angular/diagonal strength to develop these motor recruitment patterns so that we become simultaneously strong and functional. Without this, our performance suffers greatly and injury likelihood significantly increases.

The term *six degrees of freedom* refers to motion in three-dimensional space, namely the ability to move forward/backward, up/down, left/right (translation: in three perpendicular axes), combined with rotation about three perpendicular axes (yaw, pitch, roll). Because the motion within these three axes combines with the rotation about the three axes, movement gains infinite degrees of freedom. There is no limit to the variations. The motion indeed has six degrees of freedom.

Six Degrees of Freedom

- **Swaying:** Moving left and right; x-axis translation

- **Heaving:** Moving up and down; y-axis translation

- **Surging:** Moving forward and back; z-axis translation

- **Pitching:** Tilting up and down; x-axis rotation

- **Yawing:** Turning left and right; y-axis rotation

- **Rolling:** Tilting side to side; z-axis rotation

PRASARA YOGA: *Flow Beyond Thought*

x-axis translation　　　y-axis translation　　　z-axis translation

x-axis rotation　　　y-axis rotation　　　z-axis rotation

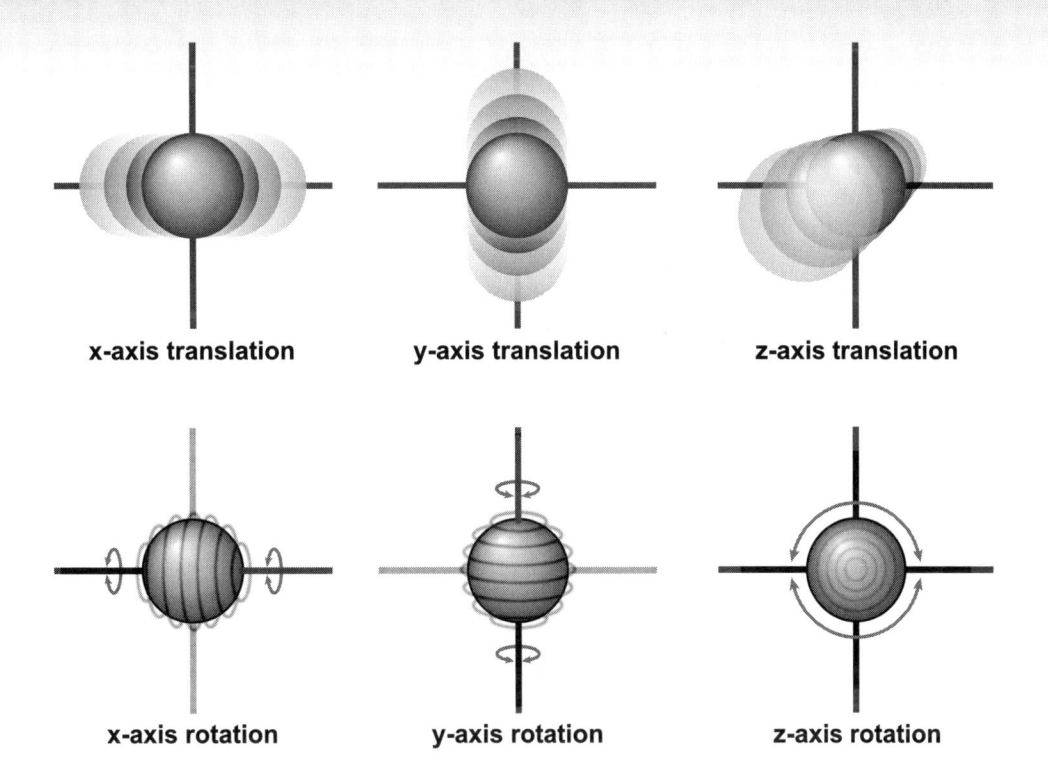

The degree to which we can flow is directly determined by the degree to which we have released restrictions to motion through the six degrees of freedom. Yoga as a result concentrates specifically on addressing this process, with individual asana targeting a particular static translation or rotation. Once breath is linked through vinyasa development, dynamic translation and rotation are targeted in prasara.

Pain-Free Mobility: What Causes Pain?

Several structures can lead to or contribute to pain in our lower back. Our intervertebral discs are incredibly versatile and strong because they need to act as shock absorption for various tasks we complete throughout the day, including lifting, stepping, and carrying. However, when we experience a sharp, surprising force (such as a fall or collision), a disc can fail. Unfortunately, when we injure a disc, it lacks the ability to properly repair itself, so recurrent pain becomes commonplace.

Compression of the cervical vertebra directly promotes cumulative joint degeneration. Our joints are lined with cartilage for protection of the joint and to absorb shock from the external world. As we age, this waxy substance in our joints degrades, as does pain-free full range of motion. After puberty, except for the mandible our joints no longer receive nutritive blood supply. The only oxygen and nutrition that our joints receive come from a fluid secretion called synovial fluid. Furthermore, over time, our joints accumulate various toxins and excess materials promoting degenerative disease and infection.

Joint Nutrition

Pain worsens the situation by conditioning one to not move the area, when immobilization is the worst possible remedy for the pain! We need joint mobility or we rob the disc of its nutrition. Basically acting like a sponge, the disc receives nutrition from physical exercise, which causes it to swell and then squeeze out fluid. However, pain can influence us to avoid physical activity, and thus prevent the much-needed nutrients from washing the area. Without nutrition washing our discs, decay begins. We are as old as our joints, so our only chance at a fountain of youth comes from drinking from the well of joint mobility.

Resolving Swelling

We need joint mobility to address the fluid exchange in our spine to reduce the swelling that happens naturally as a result of injuring a disc. The swelling itself becomes an ancillary issue, which can irritate nerves already adversely affected by the herniated disc. This in turn can cause greater pain across several structures, which further increases immobilization of the area. Regardless of the pain, regardless of how slightly it can be moved, unless a doctor advises us otherwise, we need to move the area so we can reabsorb the swelling and get to the root of the issue with further joint mobility exercise.

Rehabilitation

Our muscles, tendons, and ligaments contribute greatly to spinal alignment, agility, and structure. When not specifically moved (since they cannot be moved by simple, gross actions), the tissues can begin to adhere to each other, lose their resilience, and even tear when suddenly overloaded by resistance or contraction.

Although muscles can repair themselves rapidly, when injured they do contribute greatly to lower-back pain. Pinched or cut nerves prevent muscles from functioning, which can occur when a herniated disc presses a nerve. Furthermore, because our muscles are in continuous communication with our nervous system, fear, anger, nervousness, and so on can contract the injured muscles, leading to muscle spasm. This tension can progress, the muscles can become conditioned, and, as a result, the lower-back pain can become chronic.

Chronic Pain Creates Fear-Reactivity

If we've experienced a sprained wrist or ankle, we know the pain of soft-tissue injury. It's an immediate shock but resolves as the injury heals. However, chronic pain involves the baseline

PRASARA YOGA: *Flow Beyond Thought*

stimulation of the nervous system, which becomes embedded — or bound. It's like a low hum of information to our nervous system, which adapts and accepts the stimulation as normal.

The memory of this event may persist even after the initial irritation resolves, so when a movement similar to the initial injurious motion happens, a protective reflex of tension erupts. Over time, this baseline tension becomes stronger and stronger, creating greater and greater immobility and, subsequently, more and more intense pain.

Any type of stress or emotional distress may aggravate the area by storing the arousal of tension at our weakest link first — the site of the injury — and thereby even more confusing the site of the referred pain.

This pain may even progress to uninjured areas, which speaks to the fact that the site of pain is rarely the source. Once we adapt to pain and it becomes chronic, kinetic chains of chronic tension invariably arise.

Dynamic Mobility Training

Yoga causes an increase in the strength of ligaments and tendons in the area being trained. This is partly due to an increase in capillarisation and blood flow in the surrounding tissue, from which tendons and ligaments get all of their nutrients by diffusion (having no direct blood supply of their own).

Mobility practice is a daily requirement, whereas flexibility training is not. Mobility practice provides nutritive and lubricative fluid to wash each joint (which would not happen without movement), reversing the aging process. Flexibility training does not do this.

Dr. Nikolay Amosov, a well-respected Russian surgeon, supported the notion of mobility practice with his "1,000 moves to Heaven." Dr. Amosov completely rehabilitated from open-heart surgery with mobility practice (including with light weight movements such as in Clubbell training). Furthermore, he claimed that he reversed his aging process through this mobility practice.

Our ability to move through all six degrees of freedom is absolutely requisite to the health of our joints — and we are as old as our joints! Injuries and general wear-and-tear cause joint compression (squeezing out synovial fluid, our joint nutrition and lubrication) and create scar tissue (adhesions) and calcium deposits (joint salts) as well as rheumatoid ailments. Our mobility practice decompresses our joints, washing them with nutritive and lubricative health while breaking up adhesions and calcium deposits so we can continue to move pain free for the rest of our lives. Flexibility training cannot do this because it moves against tissue tension in one direction.

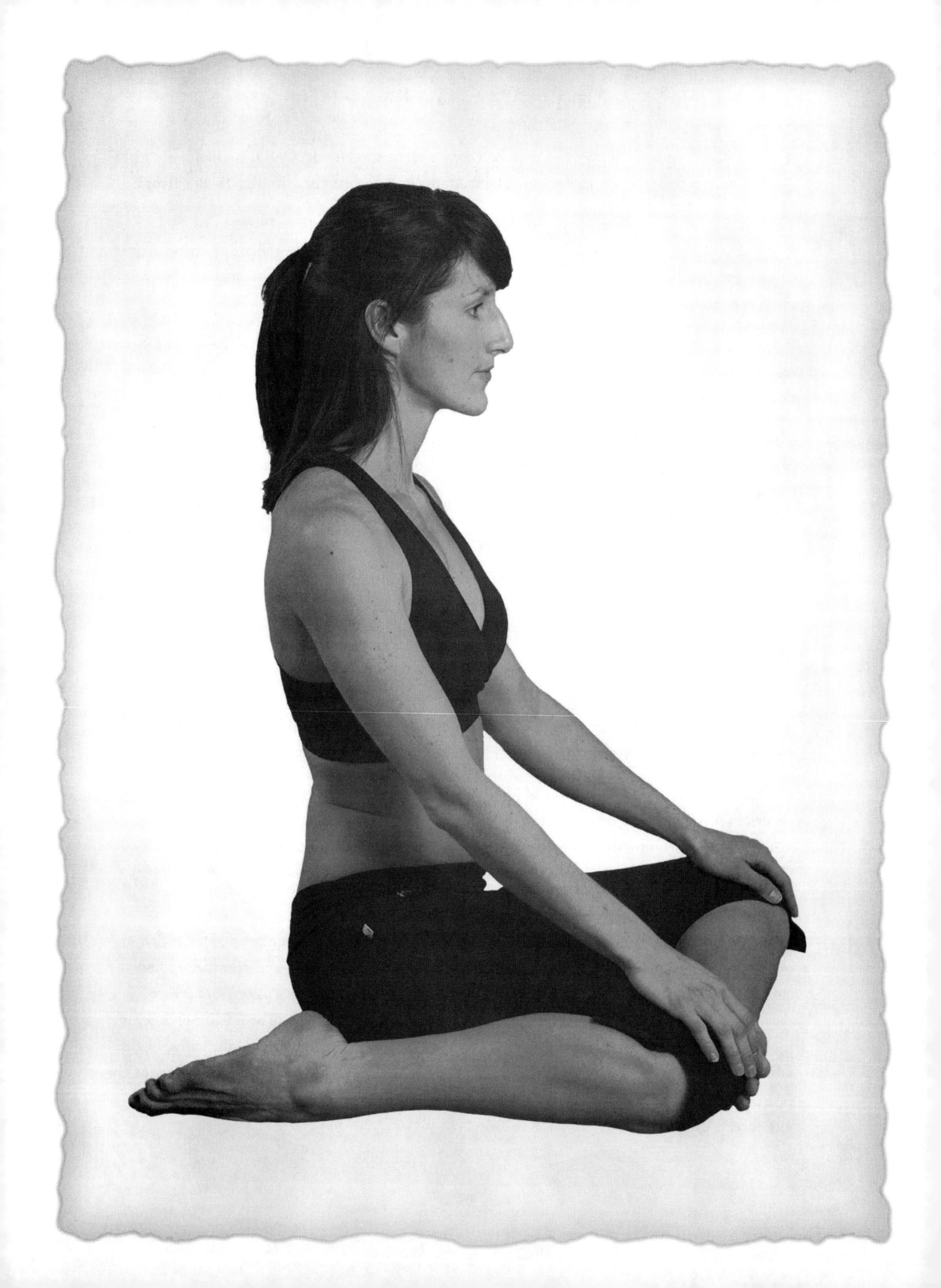

Defining Bound Flow in Exercise Physiology

When our flow is bound, it's like walking across a mud-lined river. Our feet sink and we become mired to our knees in the muck. Each step requires every ounce of effort we can muster, and all the while, people, opportunities, and life itself seem to be floating by.

Bound flow involves the pattern of knots in our myofascia (muscles and connective tissue), making it difficult to breath, stand, and sit straight and painful to move. It's difficult, painful, and energetically expensive to move with these networks of muscular tethers.

When addressing bound flow, analysis begets paralysis. We can't think our way out of a cage, especially if the cage is self-imposed and despite the fact that the bars are invisible. No amount of mental exploration enables anything regarding movement. We need to physically act in order to cast off the shackles binding our health, strength, and performance.

To free ourselves from the bondage of bound flow, we need to make the invisible bars of the cage visible. We need to identify what keeps us in and, by doing so, secure our path to liberate our health, to secure pain-free movement, and to tap into our unlimited potential.

The first thing we must do is realize that coordination, grace, poise, agility, and balance are attributes that are not learned. They are a genetic inheritance. What we learn, what we condition and make repeatable are the opposite.

The second step in our emancipation from bound flow involves understanding how we came to systematically build restraints to our flow. By learning how we build bars to a cage, we can deconstruct it and simply walk away from unhealthy, weak, poor-performance lifestyle patterns.

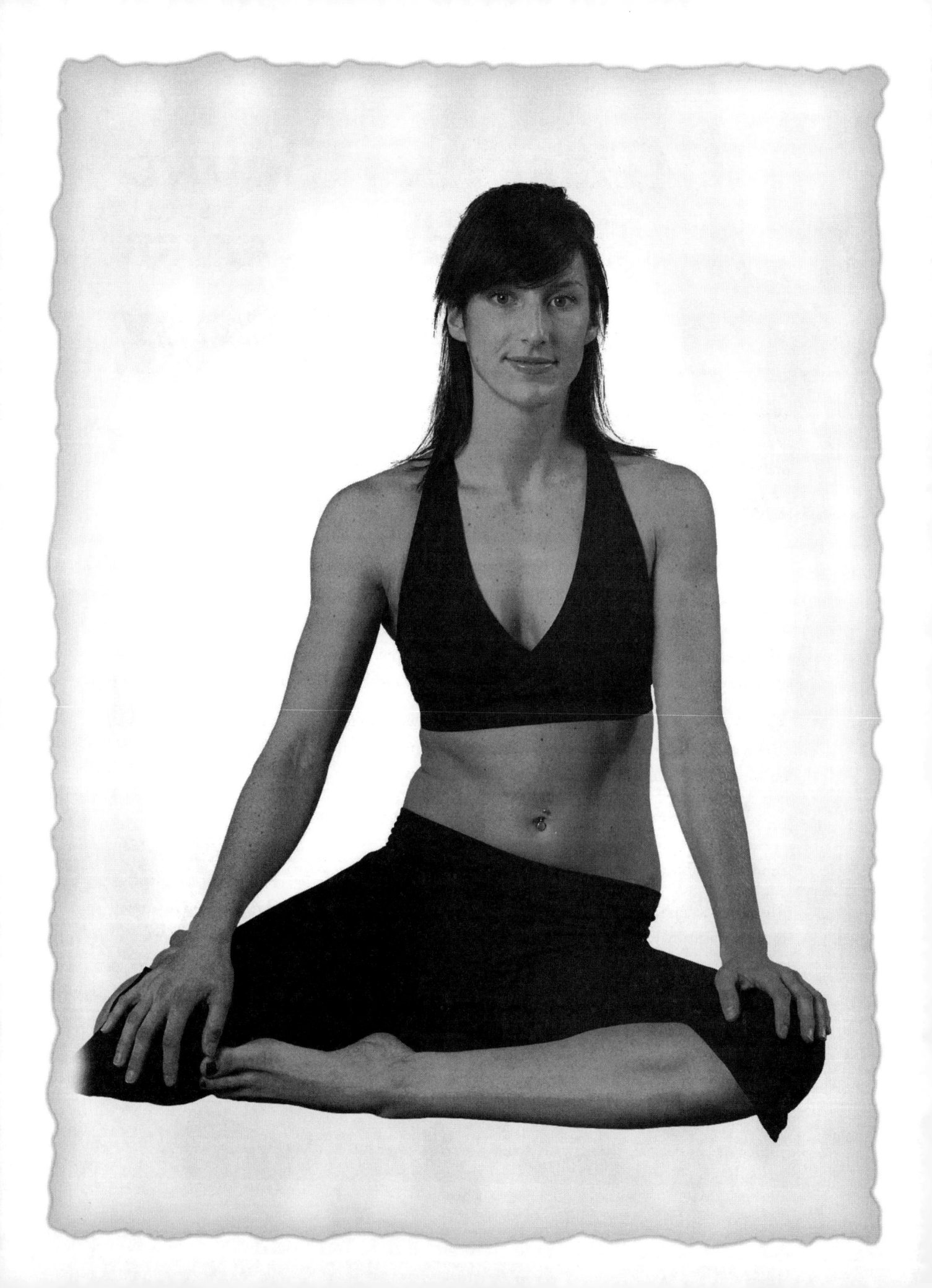

The Progressive Stages of Bound Flow

Soft tissue knows only outcomes, adaptation, and progress, so if the form (or technique) is inefficient, it produces a negative outcome, adaptation, and progression — resulting in sustained tension in that area. This obviously can happen from repetitive motion (e.g., people at a computer desk or working a foundry assembly line).

The real problem is when we suddenly and/or dramatically load a muscle that is already tense from that tension chain. A defensive stretch reflex occurs to protect the area, and we either have a muscle pull or, worse, a tear (and even worse still, the compromise of the integrity of one of our joints).

The Laws of Conditioning (*Big Book of Clubbell Training*, RMAX.tv Productions, 2003/2006) determine every action is an act of conditioning:

- **Law of Outcome:** Whatever we do produces an outcome, regardless of how we value that outcome.

- **Law of Adaptation:** Whatever we do over a period of time creates a change in us to find homeostasis, regardless of how we value that adaptation.

- **Law of Progress:** Whatever we do with continually increasing volume, intensity, density, or complexity becomes more easily repeatable, regardless of how we value the progress.

Progression refers to the body's adaptation to a certain repeated behavior. For instance, if we experience daily emotional stress such as verbal abuse and/or consistent physical abuse, we may tend to lift the shoulders and transpose the neck forward with the head downward facing. The more that this occurs, the more the body adapts by building muscle tissue and reinforcing the sustained tension in the neck, shoulders, and back.

Make no mistake about this, it is muscle building — muscle that is rock hard, highly irritable, and very inflexible with limited range of motion. This defensive bracing affects the myofascia, which becomes thick, leathery straps preventing movement. Thick, hard myofascia then forgets

PRASARA YOGA: *Flow Beyond Thought*

its natural range of motion, progressing to sensory motor amnesia. The tissues move less and less, and the sensory information coming in feels more and more vulnerable as it moves outside that very limited mobility. This bound flow then affects the structural alignment of the skeleton, which leads to a host of dangerous internal conditions.

The following chart, Wheel of Dis-Ease, helps us better understand the cycle of degeneration.

Residual muscular tension (RMT), myofascial density (MD), sensory motor amnesia (SMA), and fear-reactivity directly affect our movement capabilities and, as a result, contribute to binding our flow. As we can see from the Wheel of Dis-Ease, these stages of bound flow contribute to a vicious perpetuating cycle, a downward-spiraling feedback loop of diminishing health, strength, and performance.

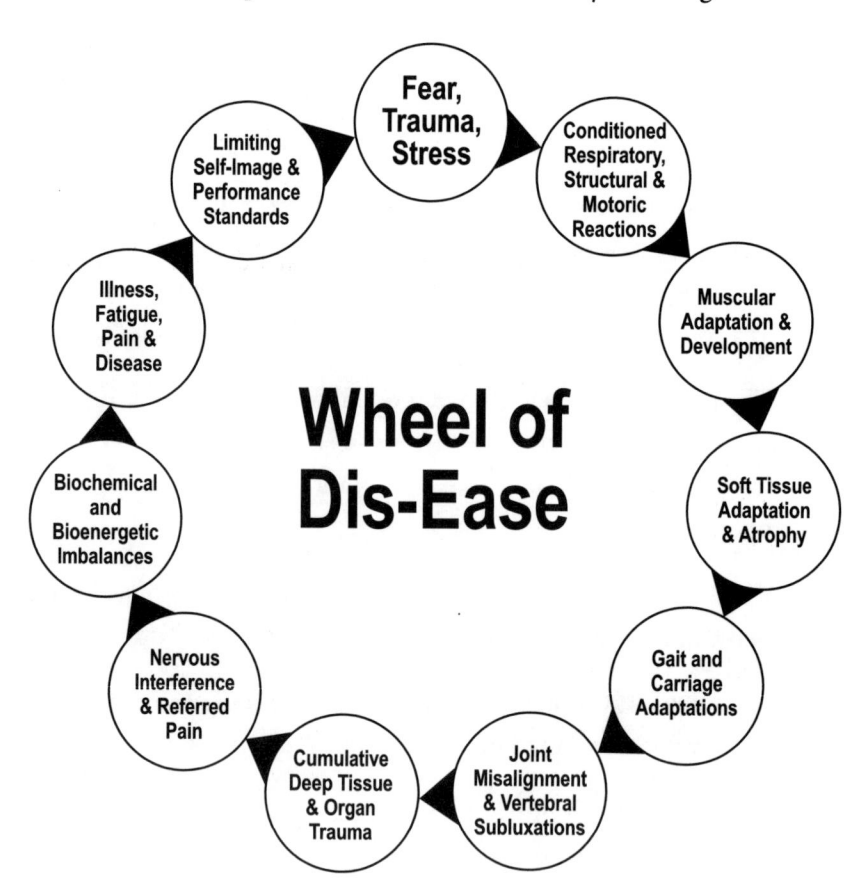

Wheel of Dis-Ease

- Fear, Trauma, Stress
- Conditioned Respiratory, Structural & Motoric Reactions
- Muscular Adaptation & Development
- Soft Tissue Adaptation & Atrophy
- Gait and Carriage Adaptations
- Joint Misalignment & Vertebral Subluxations
- Cumulative Deep Tissue & Organ Trauma
- Nervous Interference & Referred Pain
- Biochemical and Bioenergetic Imbalances
- Illness, Fatigue, Pain & Disease
- Limiting Self-Image & Performance Standards

There are four stages of flow binding, beginning with residual muscular tension and progressing to myofascial density, then to sensory motor amnesia and, finally, to fear-reactivity. Each stage progresses from the prior in a chronic loop of increasingly more bound flow.

Bound flow begins when we resist the natural course of events. This resistance is due to tension being stored in the muscles when not needed for activity.

Residual muscular tension relates to the presence of an unconsciously held partial contraction of muscles following prolonged periods of stress or activity. Residual muscular tension is the bane of every athletic training program because it interferes with rest, recovery, relaxation, and subsequent performance by disintegrating proper performance-related neurological coordination and function. It aches, limits movement capability, and eventually progresses to myofascial density.

Myofascial density represents the inelastic, leathery straps of "fascial" connective tissue surrounding our muscles caused by dehydration, excess strain, trauma, and/or insufficient movement. The body is composed of an interconnected myofascial web: a "double-bag system." (Thomas Myers, *Anatomy Trains: Myofascial Meridians for Manual and Movement Therapists*, 2001.)

The "inner bag" contains bone and cartilage, and where it "cling wraps" the bone it's called "periosteum." Over the joints it's called "joint capsule." The "outer bag" contains an electric jelly we refer to as muscle and covering it is what we call "fascia" (and other names, but let's keep this simple). Where that outer bag is tacked down to the inner bag is what we call "muscle attachments," or "insertion points." Our bones and joints "float" in a sea of continuous tension, and our bones act as compressive struts pushing outwards while this web pulls inward in a unique balance that Buckminster Fuller named tensegrity (or "integrity of tension").

Thus when we condition the tissues to hold in a particular way that is not antigravitationally efficient, the fascia lays down thick, leathery straps to hold itself in place. This then accounts for the immobility of most people who repeat any form of stress — work, family, or even training — and can result in sensory motor amnesia, and reinforce fear-reactivity. Through mobility we can reopen the density and restore fluid flow, function, and connections with the sensory motor system.

Sensory motor amnesia is a phrase coined by renowned therapist Thomas Hanna in the book *Somatics: Reawakening the Mind's Control of Movement, Flexibility, and Health*: "This is a condition in which the sensory-motor neurons of the voluntary cortex have lost some portion of their ability to control all or some of the muscles of the body. Sensory motor amnesia occurs neither as an organic lesion of the brain nor of the musculoskeletal system; it occurs as a functional deficit whereby the ability to contract a muscle group has been surrendered to sub-cortical reflexes. These reflexes will chronically contract muscles at a programmed rate — ten percent, thirty percent, sixty percent, or whatever — and the voluntary cortex is powerless to relax these muscles below that programmed rate. It has lost and forgotten the ability to do so."

In essence, SMA is a "forgotten" and "ignored" habitual pattern of muscular contraction somewhere in the body. It can have a tremendous effect on all aspects of our health, strength, fitness, and performance. For most people, this will make no "sense" until we can sense what we have lost. Basically, we don't miss what we can't remember. As we will see, there is hope. There are tools, methods, processes, and programs that will help dust off the cobwebs covering our natural grace, poise, and energy.

PRASARA YOGA: *Flow Beyond Thought*

Sensory motor amnesia (as well as RMT and MD) can progress to fear-reactivity through the avoidance syndrome. If it hurts to move in a certain way, then we consciously or unconsciously tend to avert from the pain. However, like any form of conditioning, the more we do something, the more we make that activity repeatable. And once we make that activity repeatable, we "progress."

Fear-reactivity means a trauma-created and/or -reinforced disintegration of our breathing, movement, and structural alignment. *Kinetic chains of tension* refers to a muscle-to-muscle linkage of tension, which forms from any action. Imagine when we walk, as the left leg heel impacts, a chain of tension forms up our left leg, across our pelvis, and up our right side to our right arm.

The Site Is Not the Source

Often the original source of the issue (where the impact originally embedded) creates an irradiation of tension, producing a site of injury, pain, or limited range of motion in another area. The muscles between the source and the site are a kinetic chain of tension. They are kinetic and not "potential" because although we may not be structurally moving, the muscle remains contracting (residual muscular tension).

Often health professionals treat only the various sites and never get to the source of the issue. In general, sports medicine doctors and musculoskeletal therapists are the best choices to consult when we have these issues because they look at the body as an inextricably intertwined organism.

Through movement exploration we can locate and release these chains of tension. When we address only the site, we may resolve the issue there, but it can recede to a more prior point along the chain (not always all the way back to the source). And if it is left unaddressed, a later dramatic or sudden loading may cause a new site to manifest. This is where people start to condition themselves to believe that they are injury prone.

In the deepening of our daily personal practice, we will find that we can chase the tension from site to site to source and resolve the kinetic chain of tension that way. Sometimes if we listen to our intuition, we can use the images and feelings as "satellites" to detect the source issue and go directly to it — resolving it at the beginning.

But once on the path and understanding the tools, we can do this on our own. We just cannot be attached to our expectations. We must go on our "hunches" and try not to think it out but rather draw hypotheses from inductive conclusions. This is the subtle evolution of vinyasa to prasara through daily deepening of one's personal practice.

Using incrementally sophisticated joint mobility exercises we can observe and experience restrictions in certain planes that aren't necessarily observed or experienced in conventional planes of movement. Examine the "quadrants," approaching the end range of the quadrants to determine the degrees of freedom.

PRASARA YOGA: *Flow Beyond Thought*

"For example, we can reach the terminal combined motion of right side bending and flexion by either side bending first or flexing first. This allows a quick scan to see which side lumbar joints are the restricting limiters of motion. That is, if we cannot right side bend and flex but we can left side bend and flex, then it appears that lumbar facet on the left cannot 'open.' If we reach an end range in one way but not the other, then we've identified an 'issue.' Some type of intra joint dysfunction inhibits that degree of freedom because in a healthy joint it should not matter in which direction we approach end range." (Coach Jarlo Ilano, PT, CST, RMAX International, June 2004.)

When we do find a site or a source, just remember that it is our nervous system's defensive mechanism. It is a genetic gift to have this ability to protect us when things go awry, or when movements deviate from the expected. We need to be patient and compassionate with ourselves. We need to tell the area that we appreciate the work that it did, that it fulfilled its job description and doesn't need to do anymore, and that it's now time to heal. Then we need to exhale into the area, and smile. Movement heals from that point forward.

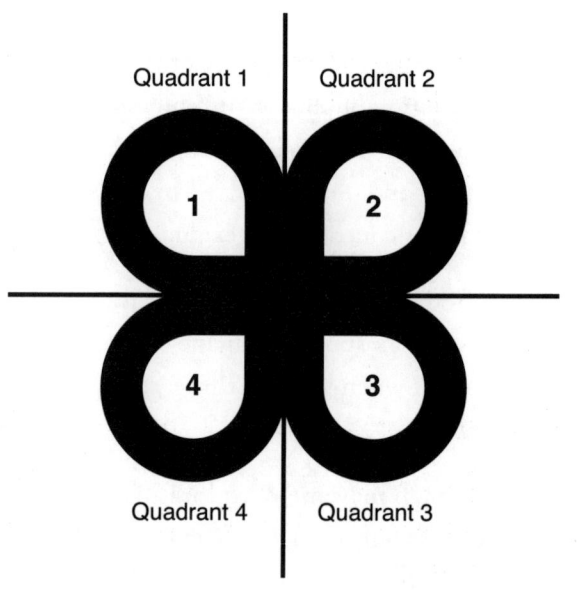

Compensatory Movement

Compensatory exercise is the concept of counter-conditioning adaptations that have led to imbalance and is determined through the six degrees of freedom.

Stored emotional insulation refers to what happens when areas remain unmoved and fear-reactivity, density, and motor amnesia creep in. Muscle atrophies, adipose accumulates, fascia thickens, synovial fluid decreases/cartilage dehydrates, and nerves/sensory organs diminish in strength. It becomes progressively more difficult to move that area — hence the emotional releases that often result from reopening it.

We Are How and What We Move!

All things are a form of conditioning! If we perform the same routine of physical exercise continuously and consistently without compensatory movement, that activity will be conditioned, adapted to, and progressed upon in an imbalanced way, causing immobility in the "opposite" direction/action. As imbalance happens, insulation/armor grows. Fear accumulates in the area to protect the imbalance, and thus begins the downward spiral of physiological deterioration.

For example, a champion in his sport may be a physical specimen in appearance. But the imbalances of his sport have resulted in a condition where his myofascia is thickened, armored, and insulated, causing him chronic pain that has led to several injuries. It is unfortunate that people frame the pain and injury as a negative. They are a positive blessing, for they call attention to the area, to the imbalance, and, most important, to the lifestyle that led to the imbalance.

Even yogi/ni can suffer this scrunching if they don't observe the yoga imperative of complementary asana. We are what, how, and when we move, just as we are what, how, and when we eat.

PRASARA YOGA: *Flow Beyond Thought*

NOT MOVING IS A FORM OF MOVING!

It is a common misperception that sitting on a couch, behind a desk, or behind the wheel is a "non-thing." These are forms of conditioning just like anything else, and we adapt to make the repetition of those events more efficient. All things require compensatory movement to balance them, including those events that are normally considered "not moving." Even the stillness of meditation is a physiological act of movement, which is why Buddhist monks embraced the rigorous exercise of yoga — so that they could endure the rigors of seated meditation.

If compensatory movement is not practiced, imbalanced adaptations will lead unerringly to pain and injury. For instance, the practice of sitting on a couch for several hours leads to the body holding forward spinal flexion, and standing and walking with effortlessness (our genetic inheritance as antigravitational creatures) become increasingly painful and injurious.

Eventually the "posture" of being seated on the couch is armored (in the same way that bodybuilding armors the body) due to the lack of a balancing compensatory movement. Once that armor is set in place, fear-reactivity protects the area from deviant movement — anything that moves the armor in a way that acts against the posture of being seated on the couch.

Emotion exists throughout our bodies, not just in our brains. We create and store emotion in the body wherever we condition, adapt, and progress in an imbalanced way — one without compensatory movement to balance a repeated event. Understanding how asana are a compensatory tool to disinhibit vinyasa and prasara flow allows us to now discuss the nature of body flow and bound flow.

The Biochemistry of the Body Flow

"Neuropeptides and their receptors thus join the brain, glands, and immune system in a network of communication between brain and body, probably representing the biochemical substrate of emotion." (Candace Pert, Ph.D., *Journal of Immunology*, 1985.)

For millennia philosophers have pondered the existence of the concept of a "mind" — an ethereal consciousness that cohabitates with our physical "body." Religious leaders, alongside the philosophers, have also pontificated on the coexistence of a spirit or soul, which they describe as a network of astral light superimposed over the physical frame.

Only a few hundred years ago, Rene Descartes received an official papal stamp of approval to work on cadavers. And in his pact with the Pope to claim no domain over the mind, the emotions, or the soul but only over the "brutal, ugly and short" life of the mortal coil, the distinction between mind and body became institutionalized in modern medicine (and for that matter the distinction between mind, emotions, body, and spirit).

However, despite the foundational work of philosophers and early scientists in understanding human existence, these crude concepts have been made obsolete in recent decades with the advent of interdisciplinary research, in particular with the establishment of the field of psychoneuroimmunology (PNI) in the mid-1980s.

PNI began as a result of the innovative work of Candace Pert, Ph.D., at the National Institutes of Health to determine the intercommunication between the brain, body, and behavior by tracing the path, nature, and operation of peptides. Peptides were referred to as "informational substances" by Francis Schmitt of MIT in 1985, relating to information theory's description of how communication networks. Dr. Pert's work helped discover that these peptides were present in the brain, the endocrine system (the glands), and the immune system (the spleen, bone marrow, and lymph nodes), and as a result stimulated synergistic collaboration between the previously independent disciplines of neuroscience, endocrinology, and immunology (which is why the accurate term for PNI was actually proposed to be **neuroimmunoendocrinology**).

PRASARA YOGA: *Flow Beyond Thought*

Dr. Pert fought a long, cold battle against old-paradigm thinking of the body as a patchwork of independent systems thought to not communicate or interact. Despite her triumph over the scientific myopia of the old paradigm, conventional wisdom still reverberates with the echo of that obsolete thinking: that the brain, behavior, and the body operate relatively independently — that there is such a thing as the mind separate from the body, which is separate from the emotions.

PNI is only 20 years old — a newborn in history. But in its short existence, it has demonstrated through rigorous scientific trials, publications, and discoveries aiding the cure and resolution of illness and disease that the mind/body/emotion distinctions are not only artificial but problematic.

What PNI has shown is that these little informational substances, these peptides, are released by the brain, the immune system, and the endocrine system to communicate with one another and with all of the bodily subsystems. And through a process of "sniffing out" and hunting down the right key-and-lock mechanism they travel throughout the entire organism, searching for the right information for the job. Endocrinologists refer to this as "action at a distance" and, as the author has stated previously regarding the myofascial system, reiterate that the site is not the source.

When those peptides lock in to the right receptors on the surface of our cells, they actually change the nature of the cell. At a cellular level, we are transformed by this communication. Release of a hormone, such as epinephrine (adrenaline), and capture throughout the body change the nature of our mood, as anyone engaged in a fight knows. Prasara yoga uses specifically personalized movements, which elicit fear so that when the neuroendocrine response occurs we do not experience biochemical shock from these hormones pumped and dumped into our system. This yoga demands courage, as anyone who has performed a Threading Bridge can attest.

Although conventional wisdom so often makes the brain and the mind synonymous, the brain is just one aspect in a trinity that makes up the information-sharing network of the nervous, endocrine, and immune systems. But even these systems themselves are not the "mind" per se. It is this ocean of free-floating information body-wide, this fleet of peptides that potentiates not just our physical state but, simultaneously, our mental and emotional states. It is this peptide network that is the body-wide mind:

"Peptides serve to weave the body's organs and systems into a single web that reacts to both internal and external environmental changes with complex, subtly orchestrated responses. Peptides are the sheet music containing the notes, phrases, and rhythms that allow the orchestra — your body — to play as an integrated entity. And the music that results is the

PRASARA YOGA: *Flow Beyond Thought*

tone or feeling that you experience subjectively as your emotions." (Candace Pert, Ph.D., *Molecules of Emotion*, p. 148.)

For thousands of years, disciplines such as yoga have had a physical practice to yoke down the physical body in order to influence the level beneath conscious awareness. And yet, until recent decades the West has branded these practices as "new agism" (even though they are, ironically, the oldest). Only recently have Western clinical hospitals included "alternative" therapeutic models to address the mental and emotional states of the patient, and since doing so have repeatedly demonstrated the dramatic therapeutic benefits in recovery, remission, and even spontaneous cures.

It is upon this absence of a distinction between mind, body, and emotions that yoga establishes its transformative physical practice. It is this emotional disposition that engenders not merely powerful, graceful physical performance but health, longevity, and a life of fulfillment and bliss.

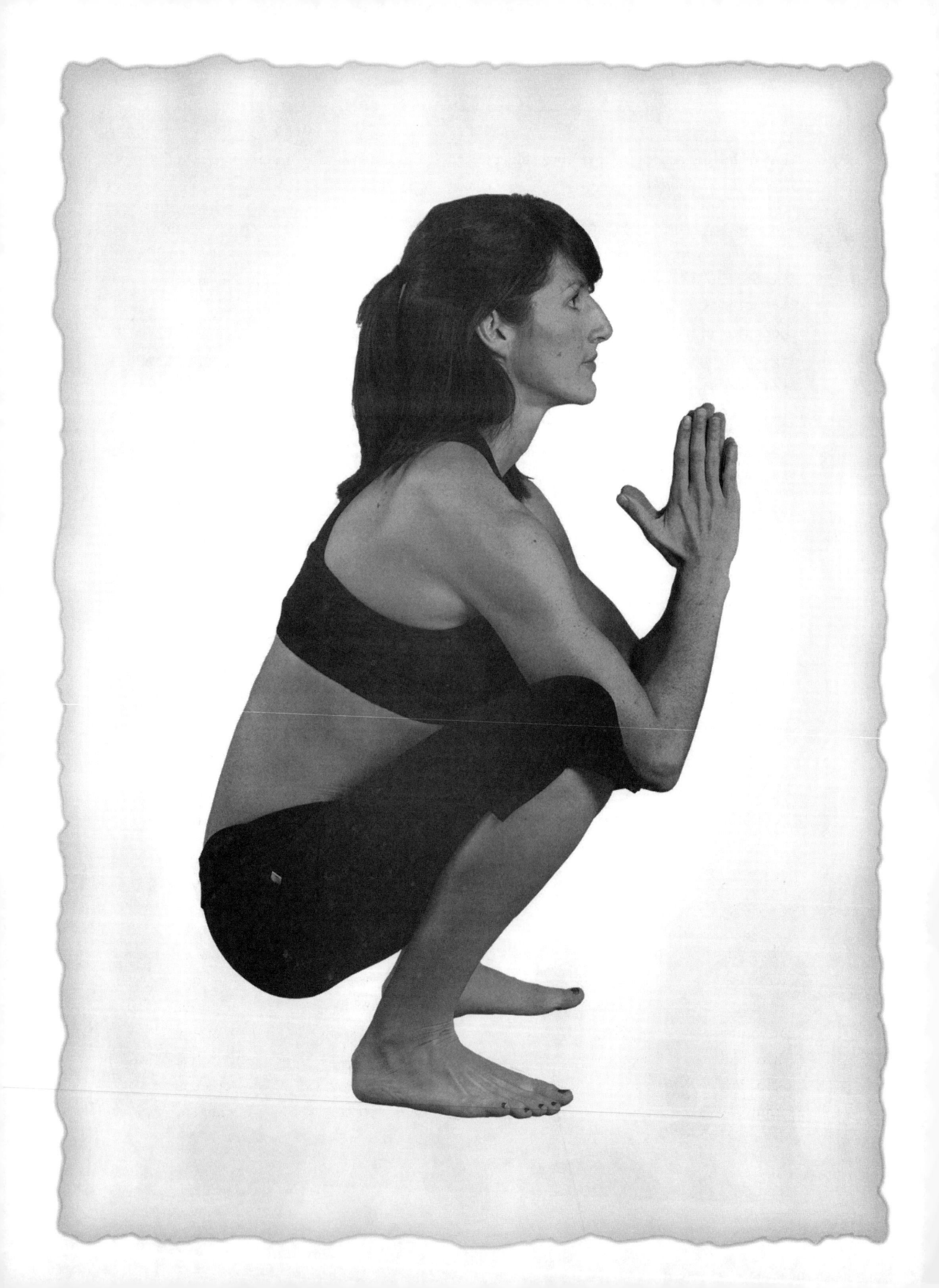

Good Vibrations

Dr. Kathleen DesMaisons, author of *Potatoes Not Prozac*, said at her Radiant Recovery® ranch, "If you try to break the capsule that holds the pain it won't work — but if you 'bathe' it, instead of 'breaking' it — it will work."

Bathing the capsule. It's so beautifully ironic that this literally happens physiologically; we bathe the joint capsules in nutritive and lubricative fluid. Muscle release relates to Dr. DesMaisons' description of bathing the capsule rather than trying to break it.

The entire universe vibrates. This is the way energy works. Muscles, too, vibrate; they have a frequency. When we hold tension, part of the muscle still holds a fixed frequency.

We can try to combat that frequency by forcing it to release, but this only reinforces it as our muscles hunker down even more defensively. Or we can "bathe the capsule" by matching the frequency through slow and smooth range of motion.

Matching the frequency requires that we revisit and match the initial tension, so at first, we'll feel tension mounting in the area. But as we move through and beyond, we match the frequency, and the muscles discharge the unnecessary vibration. It's quite an amazing mechanism.

We heal our own energy levels in our muscles through dynamic range-of-motion movement, as in our biochemistry through nutrition.

Vibration strategies have been around for a very long time, several million years as a matter of fact. Animals do this instinctively. If we alert, say, a white-tailed deer by stepping on a branch, her head pops up and her ears focus in the sound's direction. When no danger presents itself, she returns to grazing. Step on another twig and we see her spring into action, orienting her entire body toward a potential avenue of withdrawal, her muscles actively tensed. If she finds again that no danger exists, she returns to her grazing. However, this time after a couple minutes, we'll notice a very interesting phenomenon of twitching. Animals do not store fear's tension like humans can. They discharge the residual muscular tension from survival arousal (in the first instance above, autonomic, and in the second, hormonal).

Humans can obviously do this as well. And we do. There are countless rituals in various cultures to account for this, as well as just the very commonplace "Oh, just shake it off; you'll be okay." It's a part of the very fabric of being a human creature.

In *Waking the Tiger: Healing Trauma*, author Peter Levine describes how increased autonomic arousal stores tension as a positive survival strategy. Our heart rate and blood pressure increase, sending blood volume to our large muscles, our breathing rate becomes rapid and shallow, our pupils dilate. We perspire and our urination and defecation become inhibited (sometimes after "blowing the bilges" to get rid of unnecessary baggage). This arousal reflex to perceived threats or challenges can give us the necessary explosive power to run away from a saber-toothed tiger on the tundra, or to have the courage to face our most challenging pose or movement in our yoga practice.

We then become supercharged by a chemical cocktail being injected into our bloodstream: epinephrine, norepinephrine, aldosterone, endorphins, and so on. Many sport psychologists focus heavily on drawing out these chemicals through visualizations. This condition basically makes us a highly charged but chemically volatile version of ourselves.

Therein lies the difficulty. This stress arousal syndrome (SAS) was perfectly designed to bring down prey or to combat or flee from predators. But it does interfere with skillful performance. SAS decreases accuracy (by shifting blood volume from the periphery to large muscles), most obviously, but the so-called adrenal dump (for those ill prepared for the chemical download) wreaks havoc on perception, causing phenomena such as tachypsychia (or time distortion), tunnel vision, auditory exclusion (no or "selective" hearing), or short-term memory loss.

For millennia, yoga has taught how to manipulate respiration to lower autonomic arousal, such as heart rate and blood pressure. This is due primarily to the fact that only breathing has two distinct nervous pathways. So if we manipulate our breathing, we may control the arousal state of our heart rate, blood pressure, muscular tension ... autonomic arousal.

Shaking blood volume into periphery avenues may divert blood flow away from large muscles — a manual version of affecting the arousal syndrome. But it primarily serves to release stored muscular tension. This principle was taken to an extreme by the introduction of the Power Plate — a vibrational plate upon which one steps to stimulate tension to an equal frequency — minimal tonus. Researchers report instant nondeforming range of motion and even performance and strength gains after only minutes of use.

PRASARA YOGA: *Flow Beyond Thought*

Carmelo Bosco, an Italian human performance company, developed a machine comprising a vibrating metal disk upon which athletes stand to amplify vibration through the body. The effects of this machine include increased neural arousal and dramatically increased flexibility. (Chris Korfist, "The Foundation," *Intensity Magazine*, Volume 1, Issue 39, July 9, 2002.)

Vibration allows us to minimize our energy expenditure (researchers say to about 25%) while accomplishing the same if not improved performance.

It's definitely a performance inhibitor to have the "pump." Shake in between poses or flows, before and after, generally and selectively the muscles used. Gently slapping the muscles also has the same effect. It was quite disconcerting to line up against wrestlers from the former USSR as they would be violently shaking, breathing explosively, and slapping themselves. And yet, when the author first learned this technique, it was taught by a Siberian shaman right before diving with the author into the February-frozen Baltic Sea.

All movements require selective tension, so we need to focus our activation of the necessary muscles and deactivate superfluous movement and tension to maximize our performance. There are techniques we can use to discharge residual muscular tension: Something even as seemingly insignificant as wiggling the fingers during a rest pause enhances potential stamina by releasing marginal amounts of tension.

A sect of Buddhist monks residing on Japan's Mount Hiei, often referred to as the "Marathon Monks," has a unique approach to vibration training. Over a seven-year span, the *gyoja*, or "spiritual athlete," completes an arduous 1,000-day challenge, which builds to a final 100-day trot during which he runs 52.2 miles a day — twice the length of a marathon. An effortless running gait enables the individual to run these extreme distances by maximizing energy conservation while minimizing the adverse effects of stress arousal syndrome.

The direct impact isn't the greatest threat to our health, strength, and performance. The most significant hazard to our well-being has to do with how these stages of bound flow directly affect our self-image, self-confidence, and self-determination (perceived autonomy) and lead to illness, disease, and chronic conditions.

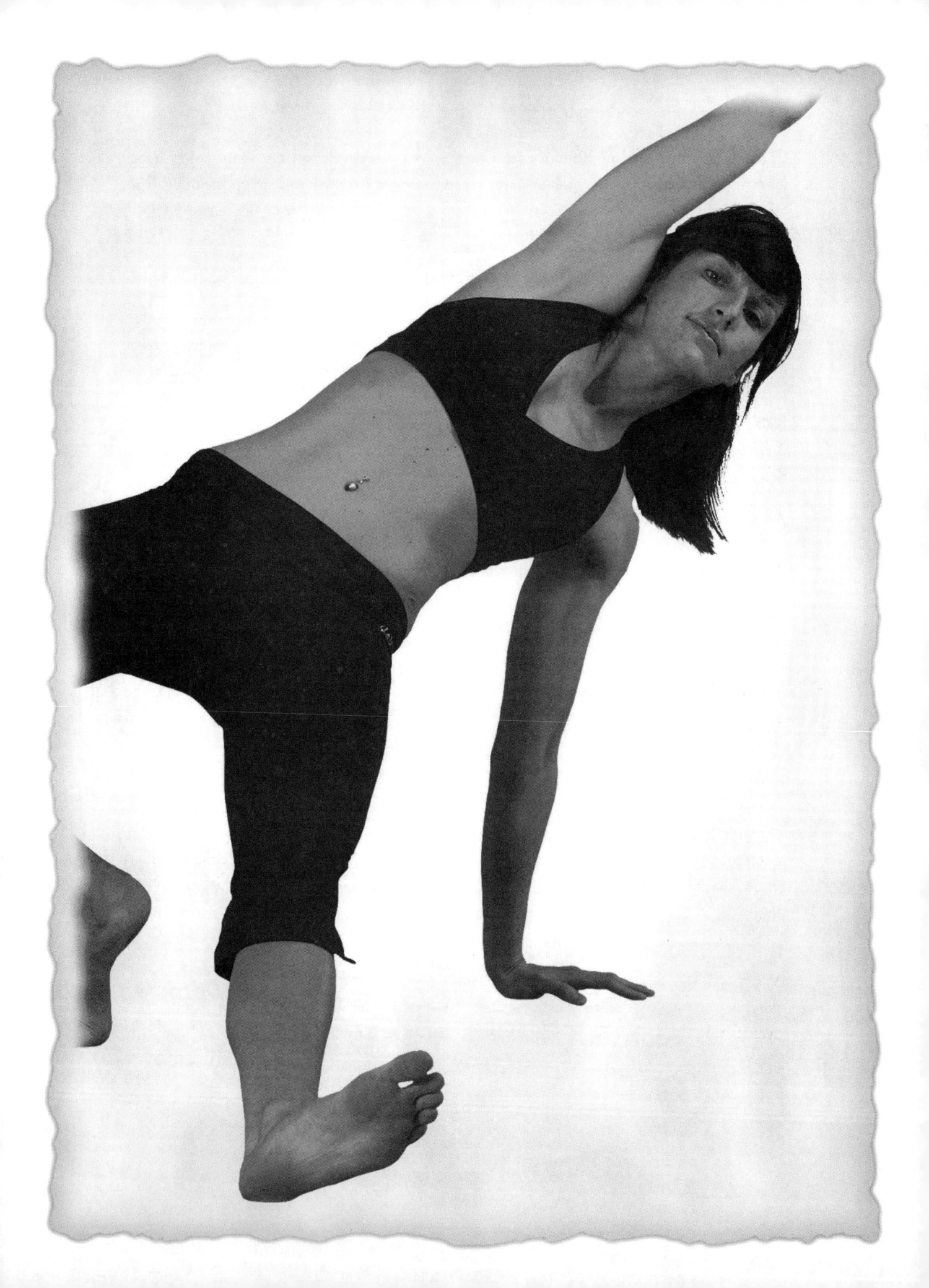

What is Fear-Reactivity?

Fear-reactivity is the nonspecific, conditioned pattern of concrete, observable behavior involving movement, breathing, and structural alignment, as opposed to the internal event, such as catastrophic thinking or emotional anxiety or panic.

Increasing the threshold of pain, such as holding an asana for an agonizing minute after minute in order to have the tension surrender, increases how well we may perform. However, doing so often means hovering on the brink of injury to stimulate the organism to adapt and progress. Progress is often the villain. Our progress can conceal our body flow if we misinterpret body flow as compilation and not distillation of performance, health, and strength.

We Are Not Our Additions

We become aroused to threats in a specific method. When we receive some sort of stimulus, we experience a specific, learned, and conditioned pattern of muscular tension, structural alignment, and respiratory behavior, which is unique to us. That tension, structure, and breathing elicits a hormonal release, sometimes slow, sometimes a fast dump. Each of those chemical brews creates an emotional feeling within us (as they are the biochemistry of emotion itself), and each of those feelings is anchored with the family of similar experiences. So when we experience the feeling of one of these we have mental impressions of similar events. Those impressions give rise to internal dialogue, evaluation of the experience, judgments … or thoughts.

We go through that process a million times a day in a fraction of a second, instantly collecting data, processing and internally representing, and then interacting with our environment. We cycle through this process each time we are exposed to stimuli.

PRASARA YOGA: *Flow Beyond Thought*

The Physical-to-Emotional-to-Mental Process

- **Stimulus:** Any novel or noxious event

- **Sensations:** Our collection of information through our senses and transmission of that signal through to the central nervous system

- **Autonomic arousal:** Heart rate, respiration, blood pressure, internal temperature, blood flow shift, and so on

- **Hormonal arousal:** Release or dump of various chemicals into the system to supercharge the system to fight or flee

- **Feelings:** Each pattern of tension, breathing, structure, and chemical blend becomes a particular feeling; one is happiness, one sadness; one is frustration, one exhilaration; one is anger, one lust.

- **Impressions:** Each feeling is categorized by similar experiences. When we have one feeling, it is anchored to similar experiences. We judge an event by the feeling we have, and those judgments categorize our experiences.

- **Thoughts:** As we make instant judgments, we react by creating inner discussion regarding our impression of what we have just experienced. Some thoughts are negative, some are positive; each, of course, is dependent on this process.

The notion that feelings come before (and create) thoughts is the first that comes to mind! But that's only the first half. The second half of that statement is our muscle tension, structural alignment, and breathing come before (create) our feelings. We've all heard the saying "If you want happiness, then smile."

But that's not the most impacting, most humbling, most numbing admission. If a dangerous stimulus elicits this process, producing a response, and if that stimulus response is conditioned, and if we adapt and progress upon that conditioning, who are we that is not a mere reaction to that stimulus? Who are we that is not that addictive compulsion to knee-jerk events?

If we are not that reflex, not that pattern of tension, not those dumped chemicals, not those phantom pains and feelings, not those impressions and not that dialogue, and not those knee-jerk reactions to those stressors, who are we?

Who we are and what we are capable of achieving lie beneath that process. Who we truly are, our natural abundance, talent, and genius, lies concealed by that conditioned fear-reactivity.

PRASARA YOGA: *Flow Beyond Thought*

Who we are is what is left when we burn away the slag that is our fears. Who we are is the slab of marble. Remove everything that is not our greatness. What remains is our flow.

Fear-reactivity refers to the conditioned reaction to stress, shock, or trauma. It embeds in each of us; no one escapes it. And in the modern world, we are beset with stressors like at no other time in history. Worse still is that we biologically cannot differentiate between an emotional/symbolic threat and an actual physical threat. If a boss or coworker is belligerent in our face, screaming at us, we become aroused (without proper training) in the same way that we would if someone held a knife to our throat.

We haven't evolved to accommodate our new postmodernistic lifestyle. We're Stone Age bodies living in a digital world. Our physiology differs not at all from when we chased down woolly mammoths and gathered berries. We still have the potential to track game and gather food, but we don't have a way to release all that stress, and we don't have a way to distinguish between true threats and false threats or distinguish between evidence and, as the anonymous acronym states, FEAR — false evidence appearing real.

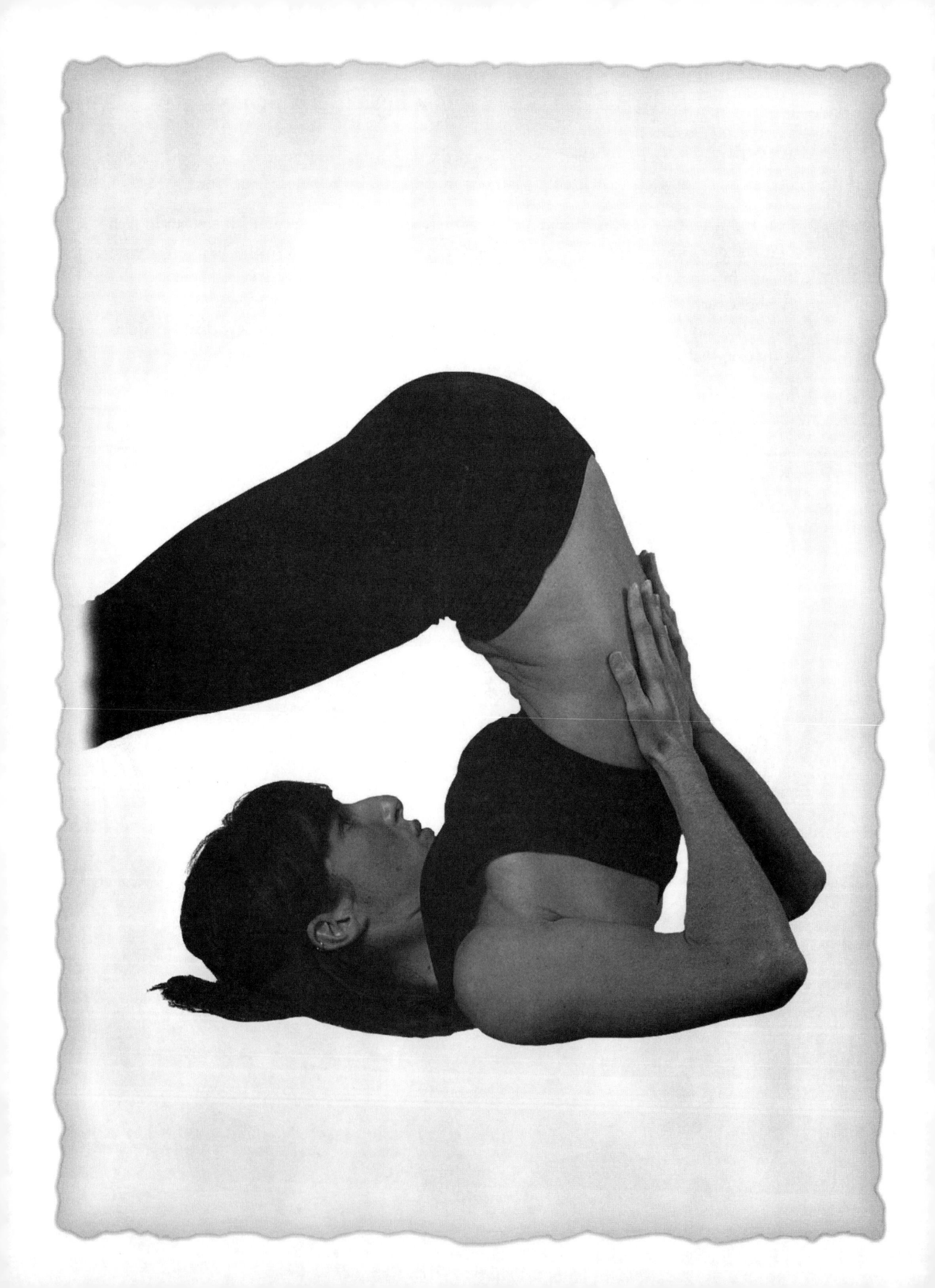

Adaptation and Progression of Fear-Reactivity

The true villain is the nature in which we learn. Any activity that is sustained we adapt to. We become more tolerant of that level of activity. This includes stress, shock, and trauma — which account for debilitating conditions such as Post-Traumatic Stress Disorder (PTSD). PSTD is traumatic stress that has not been relieved through a working through of trauma and is of sufficient severity to decrease a person's ability to function in life. (Babette Rothschild, *The Body Remembers: The Psychophysiology of Trauma and Trauma Treatment*.)

But the hazard to our lives comes from this ability of our organism to adapt to any situation. We can adapt to overeating or undereating, lethargy or liveliness, peak or valley. The more we do something, the more we adapt to make that action repeatable. The good thing about this is that we progress in strength, health, fitness, happiness, and performance. The bad thing about this is that we progress in weakness, disease, fatness, unhappiness, and poor performance. The most important thing to remember is that they are all outcomes. We choose to attach negative and positive associations to these outcomes.

However, at any time we can change them, by beginning anew, by breaking the pattern and altering our behavior. Baby steps. But before we go into how to interrupt patterns and reframe them positively, we must see the most detrimental effect fear-reactivity has on us.

At any point in our lives, there are events and situations that cause within us differing intensity and duration of stress; consider it a continuum from low to medium to high stress, depicted in the Stress Arousal Scale.

Stress Arousal Scale

- **Hypo-Arousal:** Low activation of the parasympathetic nervous system (PNS). Our breathing is easy and deep, our pulse is slow, and our skin tone is normal.

- **Low Arousal:** Low to moderate PNS activation combined with low activation of the sympathetic nervous system (SNS). Our breathing and pulse increase, though our skin color remains normal; or our skin may become pale and glisten without increasing our breathing and pulse.

- **Moderate Arousal:** Increased SNS arousal. Our skin becomes pale, our heart rate and breathing rapid.

- **High Arousal:** Dramatic increases in SNS arousal. Our heart rate accelerates, as does our respiration. Our skin becomes very pale, and we get the cold sweats.

- **Hyper-Arousal:** Dramatic increases in SNS and PNS. Though our skin stays pale, our heart rate drops off very low; or our pupils dilate and our face flushes with color; or our heart rate drops and our breathing gets shallow and rapid; or our breathing becomes very slow but our heart rate races.

However, like all things, the longer we sustain an activity, the more we adapt and progress to make that activity repeatable. In the case of stress, we become more tolerant. So in reference to the Stress Arousal Scale, our base level doesn't return to no arousal. We stay at low arousal all the time. Smaller and smaller things seem to set us off balance emotionally. And this is just the first stage. We grow even more tolerant, and moderate arousal becomes our normal state.

Like becoming tolerant to a drug, we can take higher dosages to get the original effect; that's the nature of addiction. In the case of stress, as we become more tolerant we accept more stress than before, but come to accept that as the norm, as average. Many people live with dangerous levels of stress daily because they've come to accept it as normal. Many people live with abuse (and self-abuse) because they adapted and progressed, becoming tolerant of their terrible situations.

Tolerance Affects Health, Strength, and Performance

Fear-reactivity is our nervous system's conditioned reaction to perceived dangers, pain, and trauma — often referred to as shock in cases of physical harm or accidents. That is its most extreme occurrence. Fear-reactivity also occurs under lesser forms of threat, and even when the body is not actually harmed, such as when we step down, expecting another stair where there is none, when we think something flies at our head when it is only a shadow, or when we think that we left our eye glasses at home and come to find them only a moment later on top of our head.

Prey may create fear-reactivity when stalked by predators whether or not it is caught and eaten. In the case of modern life, this can take the shape of feeling we are being followed, of anticipating an angered spouse or belligerent employer's wrath, or of anticipating embarrassment when engaged in public speaking.

Very simply, in threat, the typical escape reaction is fight, flight, or freeze. The reaction is assisted by the sympathetic branch of the autonomic nervous system: Blood flow comes strongly to the muscles of the limbs, breathing increases, heart rate increases, blood pressure increases, internal temperature increases, digestion and waste elimination are inhibited (or instantly evacuated to assist fight or flight); the system is in all-alert condition red.

After the event is over, the nervous system releases an alarm inhibitor (cortisol) and will usually return these body systems to a normal level of functioning within a few hours, days, or weeks (depending on the intensity, duration, frequency, or complexity of the stressors).

Sometimes we are unable to make sense of the threatening event — if it's too intense, lasts too long, happens too frequently, or is too complex. Our nervous system doesn't get the message that the traumatic event is over and that we have survived. The chemical signal is insufficient to halt the alarm reactions, and we become more and more aroused. We get caught in a feedback loop continuing to signal the nervous system to prepare the body. The result is we freeze in place, paralyzed to act upon the events demanding our action.

PRASARA YOGA: *Flow Beyond Thought*

The continued preparation for defensive action is at the core of the disturbing physical and psychological symptoms associated with traumatic stress. It disturbs our sleep, makes our concentration difficult, and leads to panic attacks, extreme startle reflex, a rapid or irregular heartbeat, cold sweats, hyperactivity, exhaustion, and fatigue. Psychological symptoms include anxiety, feeling unsafe, flashbacks, nightmares, avoidance of situations, thoughts and feelings that carry reminders of the traumatic event, and feeling detached from ourselves or others.

If a threat is repeated before we have had time to recover, or if we perceive ourselves as caught, the parasympathetic branch will also come into play and may even mask the sympathetic. For example, blood may flow to the center of the body as respiration decreases and our heart rate drops, while the skin becomes cold and paralysis, or tonic immobility, occurs.

Tonic immobility is loosely defined as a state of prolonged muscular contraction. Ironically that is the same definition for being "muscle bound." Tonic immobility is a state of profound motor inhibition typically elicited by a high-fear situation. Specific features include a temporary paralysis, tremors/shaking, inability to call out or scream, loss of consciousness/fainting, numbness and insensitivity to pain, and the sensation of feeling cold.

Fainting goats dropping over from loud noise, paralyzing silky sharks by grabbing their tail, the antelope that suddenly stops struggling while in the lion's jaws, the deer frozen in headlights — all exemplify tonic immobility.

The most severe case of this is PTSD, which can result from any traumatic situation in which a person's life is at risk or where he or she perceives it as such. Examples include war, surgery, rape, sudden loss, assault, abuse, and accidents. Fear-reactivity can begin from an individual event such as an accident. Or the events can be linked in chains: abuse, torture (which usually involves several incidents over time). When this trauma and the fear are not worked through at the time of occurrence, usually because adequate help, support, safety, and contact are not available, psychological and physical symptoms can develop. Typical complaints include phobias; panic attacks; night terrors; dizziness and fainting; heart palpitations; tremors; feeling paralyzed to act, speak, or decide when under stress; and other unexplainable, physical symptoms.

Everyone who faces stress of any sort suffers post-traumatic stress syndrome, differing only by slight degree. If we harbor fears, have been called defensive, are attached to issues or things, feel that we could be embarrassed, are volatile, can be easily angered or aroused, are irritable, have anxieties, experience fears or trepidations or the whole host of non-fun living, then we are subject to the above. Remember, we become tolerant — we produce outcomes, adapt, and progress. We embed fear-reactivity and it becomes more and more our baseline trait.

PRASARA YOGA: *Flow Beyond Thought*

It is fear-reactivity that must be removed. Natural synergy, harmony, and flow lie underneath the armor that we've created. We don't need that rusty suit of plate mail. We can take it off and cast it away.

Fear-reactivity is what binds our flow. To get out of the way of our natural, abundant body flow, we need to do one thing: diminish and eliminate fear-reactivity.

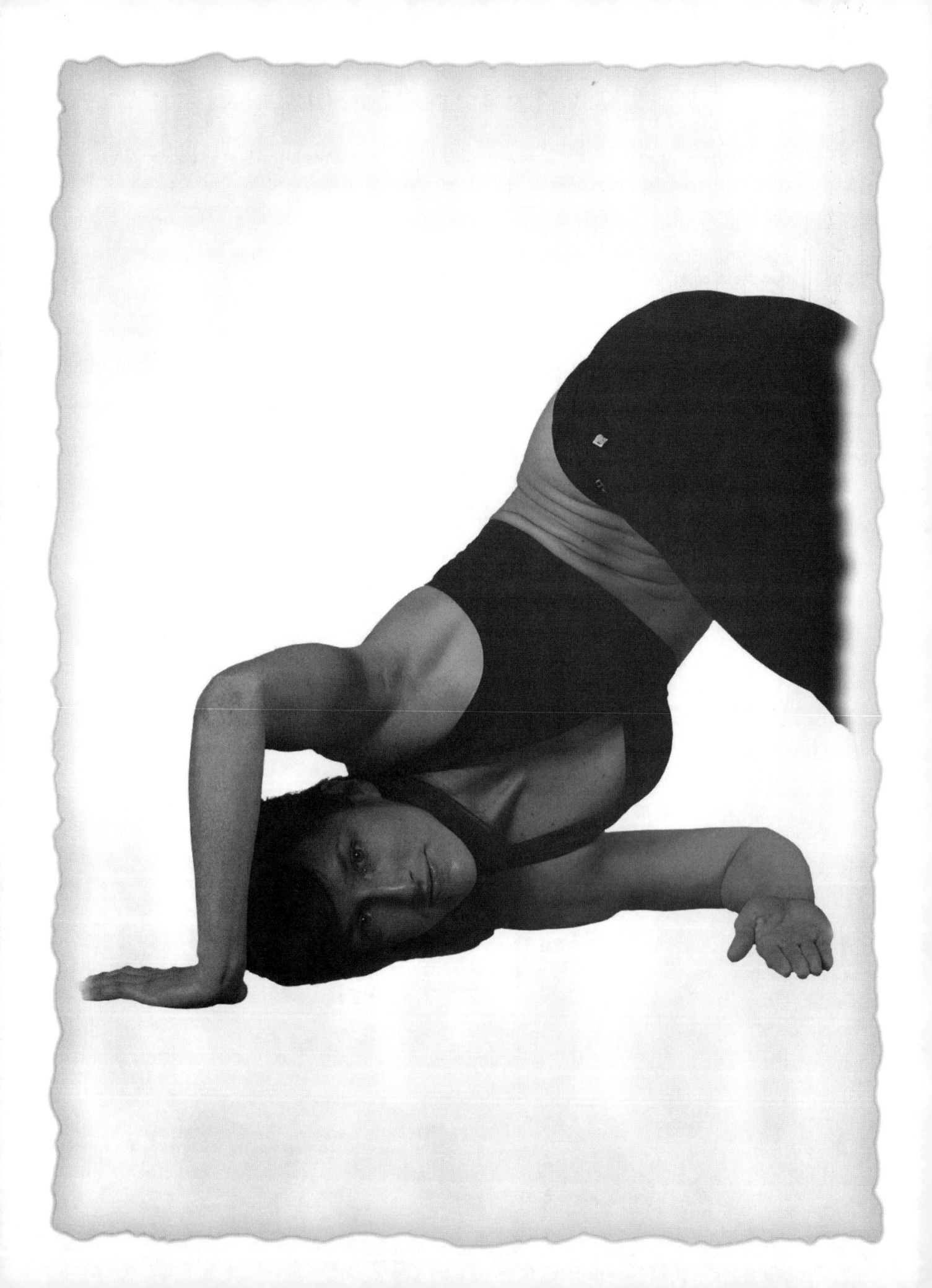

The Stress Arousal Syndrome

The stress arousal syndrome is a process of increasing alertness and mobilizing our organism. It begins with monitoring and collecting information from the inside and from the outside environment. It continues to judge and evaluate the threat level of the information, and then elicits a reflex or reaction to address the stimulus. The stress arousal syndrome comprises the following capacities, step by step:

- **Movement** involves all temporal and spatial changes in the configuration of our living body and its parts, such as breathing, eating, speaking, blood circulation, and digestion. It's our moment-to-moment state that our body evaluates.

  A state is that fleeting condition that, if repeated, we adapt to and progress upon, eventually turning it into a trait — such as the difference between being angry (a state) and being a curmudgeon (a trait). Everything is a skill, be it fatness or fitness, fear or anger, sorrow or frustration. At any time, we can choose to not reinforce a particular state by changing our behavior. We can choose which traits we cultivate. It begins with movement, the most fundamental aspect of our somatic experience.

- **Sensation** is what we receive from the exteroceptive — the five senses — and from the interoceptive — the "sixth" sense, or proprioception and vestibular sense. (Scott M. Lephart and Freddie H. Fu, *Proprioception and Neuromuscular Control in Joint Stability*.) In the next section we discuss the sixth sense, which includes pain, spatial orientation, time passage, rhythm, force/pressure, velocity/acceleration, weight/gravity, balance/equilibrium, and stabilization.

  We need to consider sensation as the information-gathering phase where we monitor what is happening within us and around us. Once we understand how we gather information, then we can begin to practice filtering or muffling the noise in order to amplify true signals. Our brain is like a satellite dish — we can direct the reception to collect critical data and to halt unessential messages to tune out

PRASARA YOGA: *Flow Beyond Thought*

the noise. Through our yoga, we learn to turn the satellite dish to find the clearest signal of crucial information.

- **Emotions** are actually divided into three substeps. To understand what emotions are, we need to realize that we often inappropriately interchange the term *feelings* for the term *emotions*. Feelings are only one subset of emotions. And because of the basic misuse of the terms, we often think that emotions lie outside of our control. Feelings are rooted concretely in our movement … the first step. And they begin with autonomic arousal:

  > Autonomic arousal provides quick mobilization of energy for vigorous movement, such as increased heart rate, blood pressure, muscular tension, respiration, core temperature, and pupil dilation.

  > Hormonal arousal washes the system with a supercharged chemical cocktail including epinephrine, norepinephrine, aldosterone, and endorphins. One major problem here has to do with the rate at which this fuel injection occurs. If we face numerous, intense, frequent, and/or complex stressors, then these chemicals are not slowly added to the system. We immediately go into red-alert survival mode, and involuntarily we throw the sluice gate wide open and dump all of these chemicals, undiluted and full strength, into our system. If we become tolerant to higher and higher levels of stress, the chemical released to halt our internal alarm system does not suffice to shut down our arousal. We fall prey to tonic immobility, as well as face Post-Traumatic Stress Disorder, chronic fatigue, and so on. (Robert M. Sapolsky, *Why Zebras Don't Get Ulcers*.) Yoga helps us regulate the positive release of this biochemistry into our system through breath control, meditation techniques, and body control.

  > Feelings are our brain's interpretation of sensory feedback from the muscles and organs that produce the reactions. Familiar emotions include joy, grief, anger, self-respect, inferiority, supersensitivity, and other conscious and unconscious experiences. We are not the feelings that erupt from arousal and hyper-arousal. Who you are lies beneath those patterns of fear-reactivity. (David H. Barlow, *Anxiety and Its Disorders*, second edition.)

- **Thoughts** are divided into two substeps:

  > Mental impressions relate to memory in that we anchor certain feelings together, and we access those related emotions when we confront a similar experience, or challenge of similar intensity, which is why in yoga we may have flashes of past suppressed, unaddressed, or unresolved events.

PRASARA YOGA: *Flow Beyond Thought*

> Self-dialogue acts as the function of the intellect, such as understanding, classifications, imagination, and memory. Thoughts erupt from feelings. Without understanding that how we feel determines our thoughts, without understanding that our thoughts, our very self-image, are a product of concrete physical actions and choices, we can become enslaved to the fear-reactivity that binds our flow. Our self-image is simply the end product of our practice.

Separating the above capacities in stress arousal syndrome is a function of literary convention only. It's nearly impossible to separate them. It follows from this interaction that detailed attention to any one capacity necessarily influences the others — the whole person and our self-image.

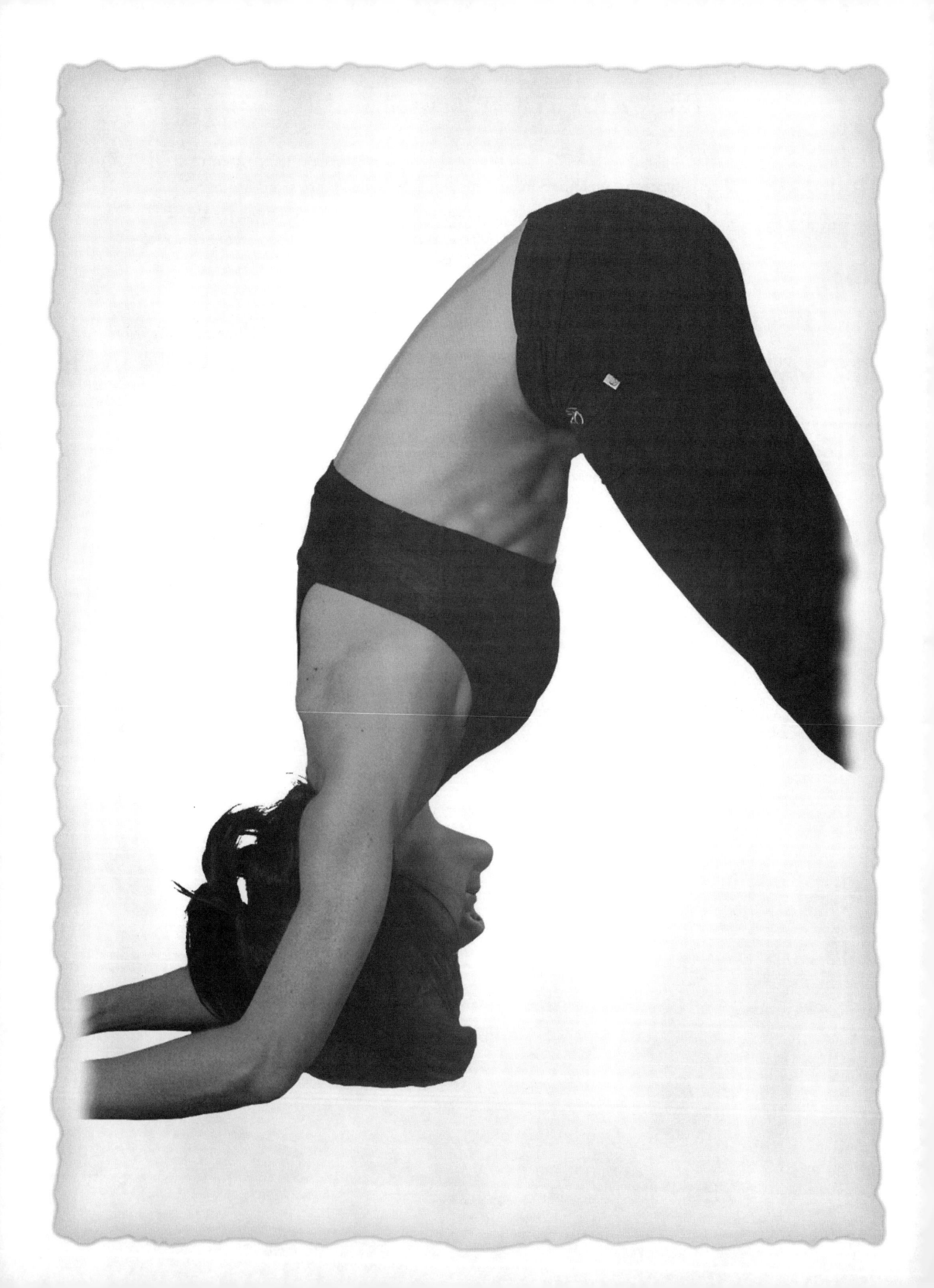

What Is the Sixth Sense?

We often can understand the exteroceptive senses — hearing, touching, seeing, tasting, and smelling. But we often discuss the sixth sense as extrasensory perception, sensing beyond the senses. Perhaps the sixth sense is not nonsense, but rather very much sensory perception: the interoceptive. Yoga in this sense is very no nonsense.

People see the nimble, uncanny, and bewildering bodily control of yogi/ni and presume them to be keepers of esoteric powers. Some develop elaborate theories and convoluted programs to develop the sixth sense. Occam's razor states, "One should not increase, beyond the necessary, the number of entities required to explain anything." In other words, all things being equal, the simplest solution among several possible solutions to a given problem is the "best" one.

What is the simplest explanation of the sixth sense and how to develop it? The best and most obvious answer is that the sixth sense is the proprioception — the refinement of bodily awareness in time and space.

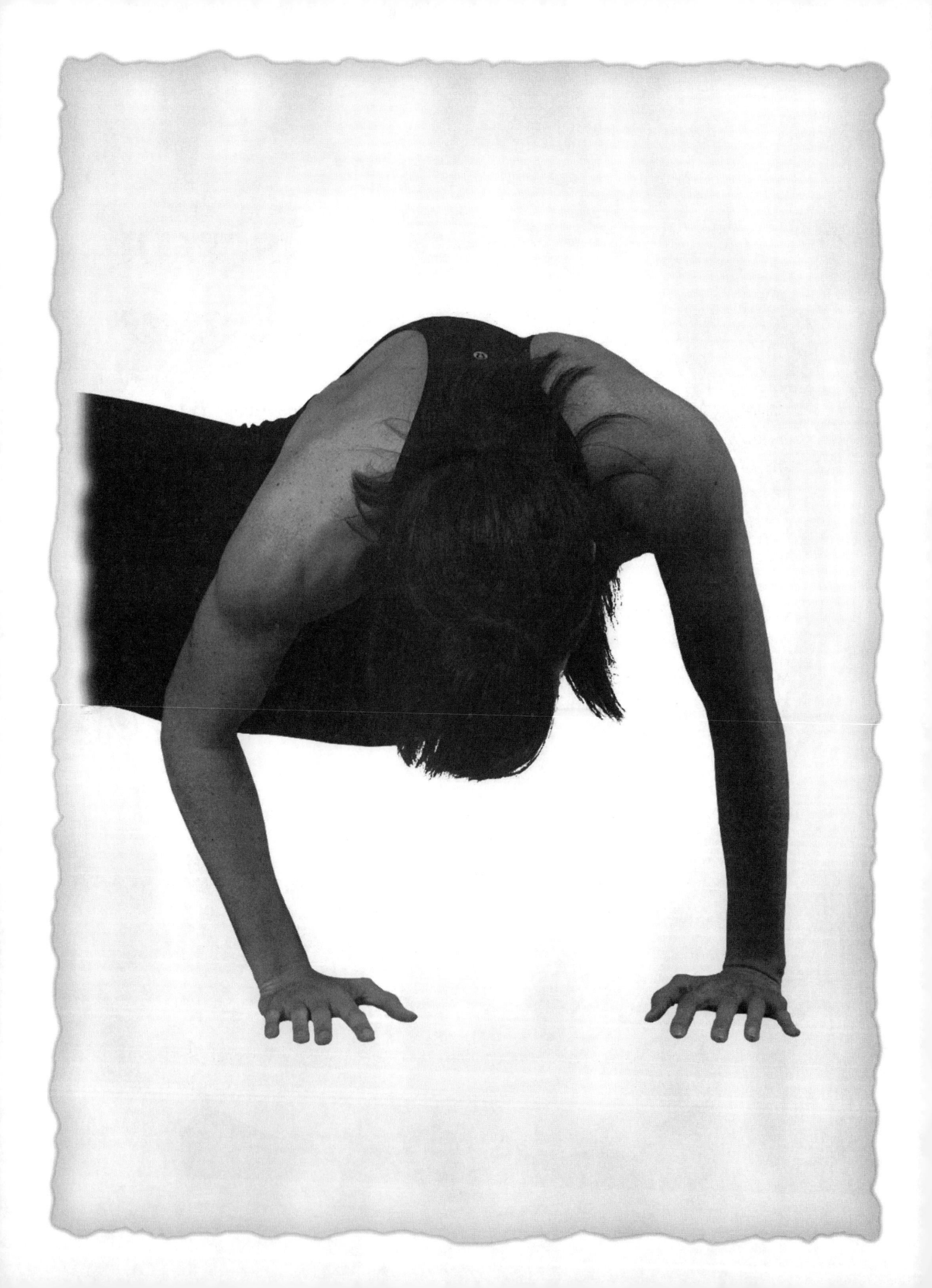

What Is Proprioception?

Scientists have remained locked in a struggle to answer this question ever since Sherrington coined the term in 1906. Proprioception, very succinctly though not very simply, involves all of those inputs that originate from the joints, muscles, tendons, and deep tissue and those signals sent to our central nervous system (CNS) for processing.

Proprioception has nothing to do with your CNS' processing of this information, nor does it have anything to do with reflexes, reactions, and responses. It merely senses and collects information. Proprioception is how we determine our place in the world because it directly assesses our muscular tensions (including our movements and respiratory control), postural equilibrium, and joint stability.

Proprioception gathers this information through special sensors in your muscles, connective tissues, and joints. Like satellite dishes dedicated to different channels, there are five different receptions:

- **Nociceptors** detect levels of pain, aches, and trauma in the body.

- **Chemoreceptors** detect changes in internal and external chemistry, such as alluded to previously with hormonal arousal in the stress arousal syndrome.

- **Electromagnetic receptors** detect changes in the electromagnetic field in which we live, and account for the host of energy work disciplines.

- **Thermoreceptors** detect changes in temperature, externally and internally.

- **Mechanoreceptors** detect three different though similar categories of information:
    > **Position sense,** also known as "joint sense," detects the position of all of your joints in three-dimensional space, including postural equilibrium, joint stability.

PRASARA YOGA: *Flow Beyond Thought*

> **Movement sense,** also known as "kinesthetic sense," detects all of the changes in velocity, direction, and angle of all of your movement.

> **Tension sense,** also known as "force sense," detects all of the levels, changes, and rates of tension in your muscles, tendons, and ligaments, as well as pressure and vibration.

All of this information is received and converted into a final common signal that is transmitted to your CNS. The sixth sense is the amalgam of all of the information transmitted to our brain to process and then decide on how to interact with the environment.

Let's consider where in the game we collect this information. Our nervous system can basically be divided into three parts. Here we look at them in reverse order from farthest from the brain to nearest:

- **Spinal cord:** The spinal cord receives the proprioceptive information.

- **Brain stem:** The brain stem receives visual (your eyes) and vestibular information — the fluid gyroscope in your inner ear that senses position, velocity, and acceleration of the head in relation to the body — and acts as an internal guidance and balance system.

- **Cerebral cortex:** The cerebral cortex processes all of the sensory information and forms an internal representation, or mental blueprint — essential information for your brain integrated into a moment-to-moment portrait of your movement in relation to your environment. What's very important to understand here is that your mental blueprint is the brain's interpretive model of your physical self-image.

Mental Blueprint and Self-Image

As a whole, these physiological data collectors create an ongoing, moment-to-moment report of our bodily status in our brain. This entire process relays very accurate information about what our body does and, more important, who we are — our self-image. Once it is communicated, our brain takes the sensory information and renders a three-dimensional portrait of ourselves in our environment. This mental blueprint changes from each moment to the next.

The sixth sense, or proprioception, is so powerful that it causes the most widespread and intense electrical activity in the brain. For example, using our mental blueprint we can differentiate between two disparate arm positions that are no greater than a mere 1.25 centimeters apart.

This mental blueprint permits us to close our eyes and touch our nose, a small task but absolutely amazing to consider. The mental blueprint is an internal sensory schema of everything in our environment.

The *APA Monitor* (Azar, 1998) reported a case where a man, because of a certain viral infection, had lost his kinesthesia — his ability to internally represent bodily position in space. Despite the fact that all of his motor functions were fine, if he was blindfolded he could not stand upright. He compensated after significant years of trial and error and managed to walk and move with relative competence. However, should anyone come into the room and turn off the lights, he will immediately fall to the floor in a heap, able to get up only if someone turns on the lights.

Without his vision this man had no frame of reference (mental blueprint) regarding where to place his hands down on the floor or how to elevate his elbow over his hand at a sufficient angle to leverage himself off the floor. When standing, deprived of vision, he had no cues on where to place his feet underneath his center of gravity, no cues on how to shift his weight, and no cues on how to maintain his balance. This was a rare case, but it definitely demonstrates the effect of just one aspect of proprioception. However, we allow the other information to compete and dominate our information collecting.

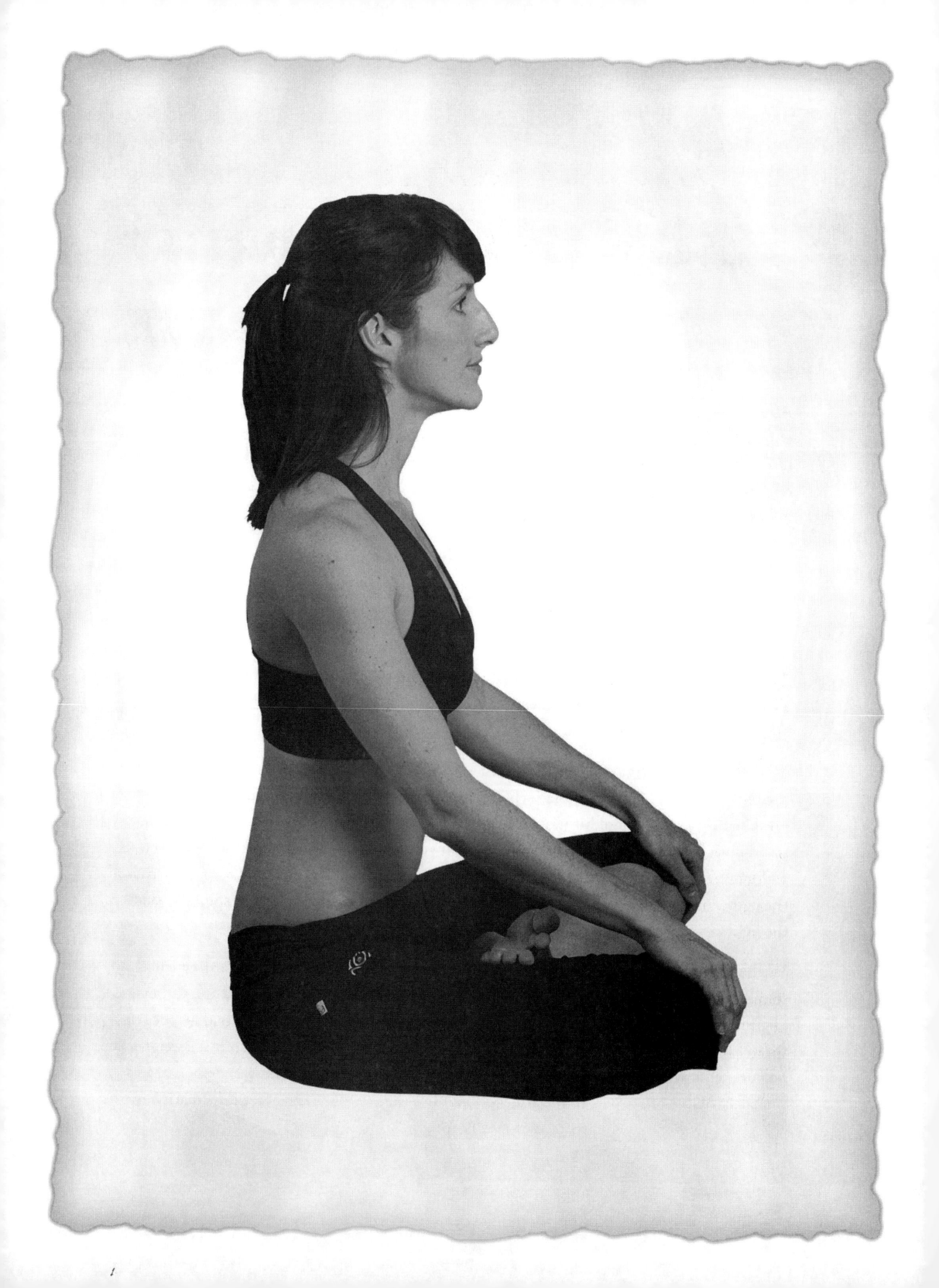

Threshold of Pain = Threshold of Performance

Pain competes for our performance. The signal that is capable of dominating all of the other channels is nociception. Pain, ache, and trauma override the other signals due to the urgency of the message to arrive at the CNS. This is simply an evolutionarily stable survival strategy. If we didn't get this information to our brains so that we could process it and do something about it immediately, we wouldn't have survived this long as a species.

The problem from a motor skill development perspective is that the presence of pain, aches, and trauma competes with our ability to release bound flow and unlock body flow. Although we may think that if we push into the pain we will achieve a particular pose or movement, we only reinforce the trauma.

We cannot stop pain, aches, and trauma, but we can unbind them so that the body can heal itself. We begin by releasing the fear-reactivity, which prevents us from accessing this healing capacity. But first we must realize that our pain, aches, and trauma compete for our ability to heal them.

As we have established, fear-reactivity is a tolerance to pain, aches, and trauma. Sustained repetition of any event produces an adaptation. That progress or addiction tolerance influences our self-image. The negative feelings and internal dialogue that result defensively lock down to protect the area or adjacent areas from future harm. This is not a negative reaction; it's our body protecting itself as part of the healing process. But avoiding the discomfort of actually moving into the area has set up artificial structures that prevent the area from healing and enabling body flow.

Pain is just information, but there is a difference between noise and signal. The noise involves all of those knotted muscles, weakened tendons and ligaments, and dry joint capsules straining under the effort of our movement.

Injury differs. An injury sends an urgent distress signal. We must learn the difference between the noise of pain and the signal of injury. Yoga helps us tune out the noise and amplify the clarity of any signals we transmit.

PRASARA YOGA: *Flow Beyond Thought*

It begins with daily deepening of one's personal practice and, more important, how we practice. Intuitive practice is a quantitative tool that will help us relearn how to qualify discomfort from injury.

Intuitive Practice

One solution to chronic pain and fear-reactivity involves distracting the nervous system through yoga practice. This conservative approach to pain management helps foster the physiological environment critical for allowing the body to heal.

In 1962, Ronald Melzack and Patrick Wall developed a new theory of pain — the gate control theory — to account for the clinically recognized importance of the mind and brain in pain perception. Though the theory primarily regards the mental issues involved in amplifying pain signals, it provides an important understanding of how yoga can be used for pain management.

The gate control theory explores the complex relationship between the central and peripheral nervous system divisions:

- **Central nervous system** (the spinal cord and the brain)
- **Peripheral nervous system** (nerves outside of the brain and spinal cord, including in the torso and extremities and lumbar spine)

The experience of pain depends upon how these two divisions interact as they process signals in different ways. With an injury, pain messages (nociception) in the damaged tissue flow along the peripheral nerves to the spine and up to the brain. But before the messages arrive at the brain, they must pass through bundles of nerves, or "gates," in the spine that shut or open if they have the right "key." When these gates are open, pain gets through and can even amplify. But when these gates are closed, pain can't arrive at the brain or be experienced.

As of yet, scientists do not understand the details of this process. However, it does yield an explanation for why yoga has been used for pain management for thousands of years.

The Peripheral Nervous System

Proprioception sends information about pain, heat, cold, and other sensory phenomena to the spine from around the body through two types of nerve fibers:

PRASARA YOGA: *Flow Beyond Thought*

- **A-delta nerve fibers** carry electrical messages to the spinal cord at a rate of approximately 40 miles per hour ("first" or "fast" pain).

- **C nerve fibers** carry electrical messages at a rate of approximately 3 miles per hour to the spinal cord ("slow" or "continuous pain").

If our child falls over and cries, or if we bump our head on something hard, rubbing the area appears to provide relief. Gate theory suggests that the activation of the "faster" A-delta fibers through pressure and touch allows the messages to reach the spine and brain first to shut the gate on the pain carried by the "slower" C fibers.

This helps explain why asana, vinyasa, and prasara are effective in self-treatment of pain. Nociceptive messages can be overridden by other signals in the manner described above. Yoga, it would then be concluded, can change a pain message due to some of these differences in nerve fibers.

Multiple factors determine how the nerve gates will manage the pain signal, such as the intensity of the pain, competition from other incoming proprioceptive messages (touch, vibration, heat, and so on), and signals coming from the brain that reprioritize the pain (cognitive pain management skills).

The message can be:

- Permitted to pass directly to the brain

- Altered before entering the brain

- Prevented from entering the brain (such as with mantra, meditation, hypnosis, and anesthesia)

THE BRAIN

When the signal arrives at the brain, the stem can muffle or stop it by releasing endorphins. With practice we can experience this in a challenging yoga session. Unfortunately, this is also how we can sometimes push too hard in practice and not realize we have caused some type of injury until afterwards. We need the governor of intuitive practice to control how much we exert and for how long we persist.

When we injure ourselves acutely, like breaking a bone or being sharply cut, the A-delta nerve fibers open the gate wide and send the message to the thalamus and cerebral cortex, where all of our "thinking" takes place, so that we can act quickly on the site of the acute injury.

PRASARA YOGA: *Flow Beyond Thought*

However, the typical aching, cramping, or dull chronic pains we experience travel along the slow-moving C-fiber nerve path to the hypothalamus (which releases stress hormones) and limbic system (which processes emotions). Understanding this, we can appreciate why chronic aches and pains throughout the body so often associate with depression, stress, and anxiety because the messages pass through the same parts of our brain that control these emotions and feelings.

In addition to our physical practice, how we frame our mental attitude about our practice controls whether the nerve gates to pain open or close. We have all experienced a time when stress and anxiety have actually amplified physical pain. The reverse, however, is true as well. We can prevent or muffle pain through our mental attitude.

Considering all of these factors, when a yoga teacher says "Go to the edge," this is what he or she means.

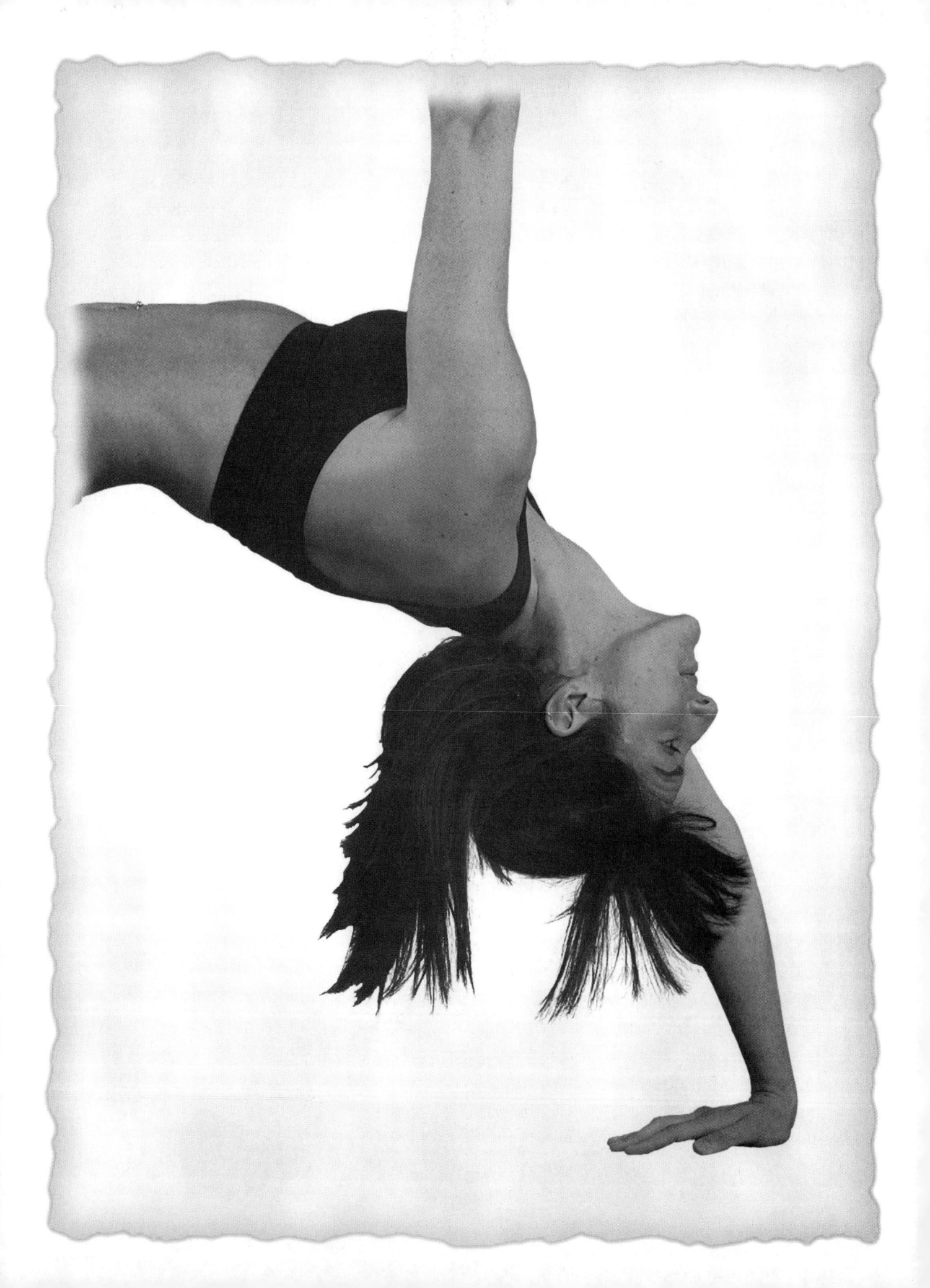

Intuitive Practice: Going to the Edge

Immobility often involves progressive stiffness. As you avoid painful movement, your body adapts to the tension protecting the area from the painful movement. It then progresses and develops strength to maintain an immobilized state. Therefore, sometimes we must move through a range of motion as long as we can tolerate the discomfort.

We live in a subjective world, flooded with changing emotions, fluctuating energy levels, mysterious pains, and surprise stressors.

Everyone at some time in their lives has experienced fluctuations of some kind among common variables: performing the same pose twice can seem harder, running the same distance can seem longer, resting the same duration can seem shorter, and so on. The subjective experience differs from one moment to the next. The sum total of stress in our lives at a particular point determines if the gates are open or closed to pain, and how much anxiety or elation we experience.

Before we are able to apply effort in a pose, we must first have the proper form sufficient to "hold" the discomfort we are going to experience, the discomfort necessary to release residual tension, myofascial density, and fear-reactivity and awaken from sensory motor amnesia:

- **Rating of Perceived Technique (RPT):** On a scale of 1–10 (1 being very sloppy and 10 being the best form you could ever do), we need an 8 (extremely good) in technique before we start to apply effort or experience discomfort.

- **Rating of Perceived Discomfort (RPD):** On a scale of 1–10 (1 being insignificant annoyance and 10 being intolerable agony), our "edge" is a 3 (uncomfortable). We need to go to that edge, but no farther.

- **Rating of Perceived Effort (RPE):** Our edge takes effort. How much effort we apply determines whether or not we develop and whether or not we become injured. On a scale of 1–10 (1 being incredibly easy and 10 being the hardest you've ever exerted yourself), going to our edge is a 6 (very hard).

PRASARA YOGA: *Flow Beyond Thought*

So when we are exploring an asana, vinyasa, or prasara, we first need a technique of at least an 8 before we can apply effort of 6 and experience a discomfort level of 3.

Some feel off-put by quantitative evaluations of the subjective experience. However, we must remember that when we are beginning a new pose or movement, or beginning yoga altogether, we often have lost touch, or become disconnected from that internal experience of the pose or movement. Therein lies the problem. Intuitive practice gives us a tool to transition from the externalized experience of *doing* yoga to the internalized experience of *being* yoga.

Calisthenics Versus Yoga

Bodyweight exercise, historically known as calisthenics, emphasizes strength, endurance, and flexibility. Calisthenics use the weight of the body as a form of resistance to condition the body. Bodyweight exercises must have technical simplicity so that athletes may immediately execute the skill.

Yoga, sometimes historically referred to as self-gymnastics or acrobatics, emphasizes agility, coordination, and balance. Yoga must have technical sophistication so that we may sufficiently unlock our flow. As in its incipience, the primary goal is flow-state, or Samadhi.

Yoga asana, vinyasa, and prasara, once technically developed, may be able to be used as bodyweight exercise, but the reverse is not true. This is because bodyweight exercise lacks the sophistication necessary to unbind your flow. That is, until we have internalized the essence of yoga, that in all human movement, we are doing yoga. Then, any movement becomes an opportunity for us to release bound flow and unlock bound flow.

But to do this, the method with which the movement is applied determines if it is merely exercise for strength and conditioning or if it is yoga, specifically crafted as a physical vehicle toward flow-state.

To distinguish between the two methods, observe the protocol: Bodyweight exercise is viewed as training, and yoga is viewed as practice. *Training* refers to repetition for increasing attributes such as strength, stamina, endurance, and flexibility. *Practice* refers to technical development to recover, coordinate, and refine a skill so that the person gains unconscious competence (the autonomic stage of development).

Bodyweight exercise movements are so basic that it appears that little practice is required. As a result they can be used immediately for training. However, as soon as effort and persistence are inserted into these movements, because training is the objective, the form breaks down. When form deteriorates, unintentional and undesirable training effects embed somewhere in the body. Because the focus is training, the bodyweight exercise cannot "hold" effort and persistence, like the yoga asana. Note here that we can mutate a yoga asana such as Plank

PRASARA YOGA: *Flow Beyond Thought*

Pose into a bodyweight exercise if our focus is on creating a training effect. When we do this, we prioritize the training effect (increased strength, endurance, stamina, and so on) over deepening form. Then, it is no longer yoga.

Yoga augments the quality of our physicality by integrating our breathing, movement, and structure. Attributes such as strength, endurance, and stamina are natural by-products of our practice, but they are not the focus, nor is physique, the physical beauty of our shape. If attributes or appearance becomes the focus, we lose our yoga.

The protocol that distinguishes yoga is practice. Once we have internalized how to practice through daily deepening of our personal practice, then we can expand our practice to all things.

Core Activation Inside Out

Critical to yoga is our "core." Movement in the three-dimensional world necessarily involves rotational and angular/diagonal action. The stability of our trunk, therefore, can be found only through improvement of our attention to core mobility.

Our abdominal muscles involve both internal and external portions, though most fitness approaches fixate on the external: the rectus abdominus (our six-pack) and the external obliques. If we lie down on the floor, we can feel the rectus abdominus flex the spinal column forward 30 degrees. If we move beyond this, we're actually engaging the hip flexors and going beyond the nature of core activation. Our trunk rotates primarily under the power of the external obliques.

In yoga, our focus is on the inner unit: the transversus abdominus and the lumbar multifidus. These tissues exist underneath the external abdominals and control our respiration and our structural alignment, contributing to our total health, performance, and strength.

Inner to Outer Unit Core Activation

Nikolai Bogduk and Lance Twomey published *Clinical Anatomy of the Lumbar Spine* in 1987. They were the first to introduce clinical observations of the abdominal and back muscles coordinating as a "functional unit."

What Is the Outer Unit?

In 1999, Australian scientists C. Richardson, G. Jull, P. Hodges, and J. Hides published *Therapeutic Exercise for Spinal Segmental Stabilization in Low Back Pain*. Within, they first coined the term *inner unit*, describing how the deep abdominal wall works synergistically with the outer unit — the conventional targets of fitness: rectus abdominus, obliquus externus abdominis, and psoas.

PRASARA YOGA: *Flow Beyond Thought*

What Is the Inner Unit?

Paul Chek explains the inner unit as "describing the functional synergy between the transversus abdominis and posterior fibers of the obliquus internus abdominis, pelvic floor muscles, multifidus and lumbar portions of the longisssimus and iliocostalis, as well as the diaphragm." ("The Inner Unit: A New Frontier In Abdominal Training," *IAAF Technical Quarterly: New Studies in Athletics*, April 1999.)

We can consider the inner unit to be the myofascia stabilizing and protecting our internal architecture, but also the bridge to controlling breathing and, as a result, our autonomic nervous system. The correct firing of the inner unit and its effective recruitment not only affects our spinal stabilization so that our prime movers can get in there and get the job done, but it also affects our ability to breath and move.

Breath links both aspects of the nervous system: autonomic and voluntary. When a particular local site manifests an issue, moving through it, around it, or with it may cause breath holding and bracing — an involuntary protective fear reflex to keep the injured area from further trauma.

This bracing serves no purpose in healing. It can only serve to reinforce the potential for ongoing problems in the local site and reinforce the chain of density, tension, or injury by forcefully maintaining the body's focus on the local site. This is why "power breathing" and "high tension" techniques may be able to increase tension locally and globally for the short term but only result in eventual injury. This is additionally why powerlifters (whether recreational or competitive, with bodyweight or weighted equipment) are, if not immediately then eventually, riddled with aches, pains, injuries, and structure dysfunctions.

Because voluntary exhalation is a relaxation trigger for the entire system, exhaling through a discovered local tension can cause the tissue to relax. Therefore, we must use active exhalation through perceived effort, discomfort, or fear to release the local issue so that the structure can reorganize in its innate, normal, pain-free form.

Dangers of Fitness Core Training

As a result of the conventional fixation on the crunch/sit-up–style abdominal exercise, a culture of postural distortion is readily observable, even if we only look at any gym, and most actors, models, personal trainers, martial artists, physical therapists, and celebrity coaches. We see chronic forward spinal flexion of forward transposed neck; sunken chest (and of course compensatory overdeveloped pecs); distended, overdeveloped abdominal wall; and posterior-tilted pelvis (accompanied by a "fanny pack" of lower-back tension).

PRASARA YOGA: *Flow Beyond Thought*

The overemphasis of outer unit abdominal work pulls the chest downward and the neck forward and pulls the hip flexors tight, creating the collapsed posture so prominent in today's fitness industry. These imbalances create inherent postural weaknesses, especially in the lower back and the shoulders, and have significantly contributed to the high prevalence of lower-back and shoulder injuries in patients appearing in physical therapy clinics.

But even farther along on the Wheel of Dis-Ease are the chronic implications of postural distortions. Postural distortions progress into cumulative deep-tissue and organ trauma, nervous interference and pain, biochemical and bioenergetic imbalances, illness, fatigue, and disease.

The Firing Sequence of Inner to Outer Unit

Chek points out in the article "The Inner Unit: A New Frontier In Abdominal Training" that research has shown that the inner unit exists under a different neurological control than the outer unit. Fitness training focuses on the outer unit to the exclusion of the inner unit. This fixation on the six-pack creates an improper firing sequence for the core, which promotes ineffective breathing patterns, poor posture, postural distortions, and joint instability.

When we miswire the inner unit through poor practices, exerting any type of effort can predispose the spine to force that it cannot stabilize and/or absorb. This often results in sacroiliac joint and spinal injury. When we allow the wiring to fire naturally, we seldom experience injury, even under intense stress.

Fitness Core Training Versus Core Activation

The current emphasis of core training of this genre involves postural stabilization in isolated positions through very simplistic and highly specific (to the activity or injury) therapeutic exercise. However, this doesn't address how an ineffective inner unit recruitment and firing sequence affects the performance of athletic and vocational tasks.

Exercises are useful for training the inner unit because they teach the following:

- The correct breathing patterns in yoga allow optimal recruitment of the core during dynamic movement.

- The rotation and compression in yoga encourage inner unit recruitment while relieving unnecessary tension in the outer unit structures.

Core activation in yoga addresses movement outside of the contexts of traditional therapeutic exercise for postural alignment to alleviate lower-back pain. Yoga basically involves using the breath to relax into challenging physical conditions.

PRASARA YOGA: *Flow Beyond Thought*

If we incrementally sophisticate from asana to vinyasa to prasara (and back to asana), we can prevent and/or release unnecessary outer unit muscle tension while maintaining effective inner unit tension to safely stabilize the structure through the motion. This allows us to keep the correct, natural firing sequence of inner to outer.

Chek offered the metaphor of a pirate ship to describe the inner-outer unit synergy. He compares the inner unit to the cables directly holding the mast upright and the outer unit to the cables mounted to the ends of the ship. The result is a tensegrity structure — a sere of continuous tensions pulling in, with the compressive struts of the mast pushing out. Without correct inner unit stabilization, the mast will buckle under the strain of wild winds filling the sails.

Let's discuss the most important point in this sailboat metaphor: the wind in the sails, or our breath. Many times we condition breathing techniques that do not sync up with structural stabilization and movement efficiency. We actually defeat core stabilization by breathing in a way that doesn't sync with the architecture of our structure and movement. Fortunately, asana teaches us how to use our breath to balance strength and surrender in a pose; and vinyasa teaches us how to resync our breath in motion between poses.

Breathing should derive from structural compression/expansion and inner unit activation — basically, exhalation on compression and activation, inhalation on expansion and deactivation. When this process is done correctly, the total performance output is greater than any of the sum of its parts due to the synergistic effect of natural integration of breathing, movement, and structure.

Now, although this is the proper firing sequence, in challenging conditions we cannot just adopt this ability to breathe in flow. We must first discipline our breath to counter-condition prior dysfunctional breathing patterns that have been destabilizing our core. We discuss this in the next section.

Chek gives an exercise example of the musculoskeletal dynamics of inner-outer unit synergy: "Almost in synchrony with the thought, 'pick up the weights from the floor,' the brain activates the inner unit, contracting the multifidus and drawing in the transversus abdominis. This tightens the thoraco-lumbar fascia in a weight belt-like fashion. Just as this is happening, there is simultaneous activation of the diaphragm above and the pelvic floor below. The effect is to encapsulate the internal organs as they are compressed by the transversus abdominis. This process creates both stiffness of the trunk and stabilizes the joints of the pelvis, spine and rib cage, allowing effective force transfer from the leg musculature, trunk and large prime movers of the back and arms to the dumbbells." ("The Inner Unit: A New Frontier In Abdominal Training.")

PRASARA YOGA: *Flow Beyond Thought*

These breathing patterns would naturally occur if not inhibited by overuse of ineffective breathing instruction, performance anxiety, trauma, and tension. Inner unit recruitment and firing sequence produce powerful breathing patterns if we release fear-reactivity and allow natural breathing to occur.

Like a String of Pearls

Our spine should move like a string of pearls. This is not in conflict with traditional therapeutic exercise for postural alignment. On the contrary, it involves movement outside of the context of maintaining an "upright posture." Life is so dynamic, and our movement capability reflects this.

In Chek's metaphor, the shipmates busy themselves with appropriate tension on the cables and ropes to secure the mast — both the small segmental stabilizers and the large movers. Without a correct timing of the inner and outer muscular units or by overuse/hypertension of one direction of cables, the mast's alignment is disrupted. Smooth sailing becomes impossible.

However, the metaphor falls short in addressing that in our body the mast, our spine, moves, bends, and twists and, ultimately, behaves like a string of pearls. Being able to expand and collapse the sails when moving, bending, and twisting while effectively stabilizing the mast is our goal in yoga.

We must rewire our unit firing so that we move from inner to outer. We can do this through our breathing, but we must do so in a context-specific developmental pattern.

If we take the natural firing sequence and augment it, we powerfully integrate our breathing, movement, and structure in all our activities all the time. This is the key to flow-state and the precursor to understanding the Breath Mastery Scale.

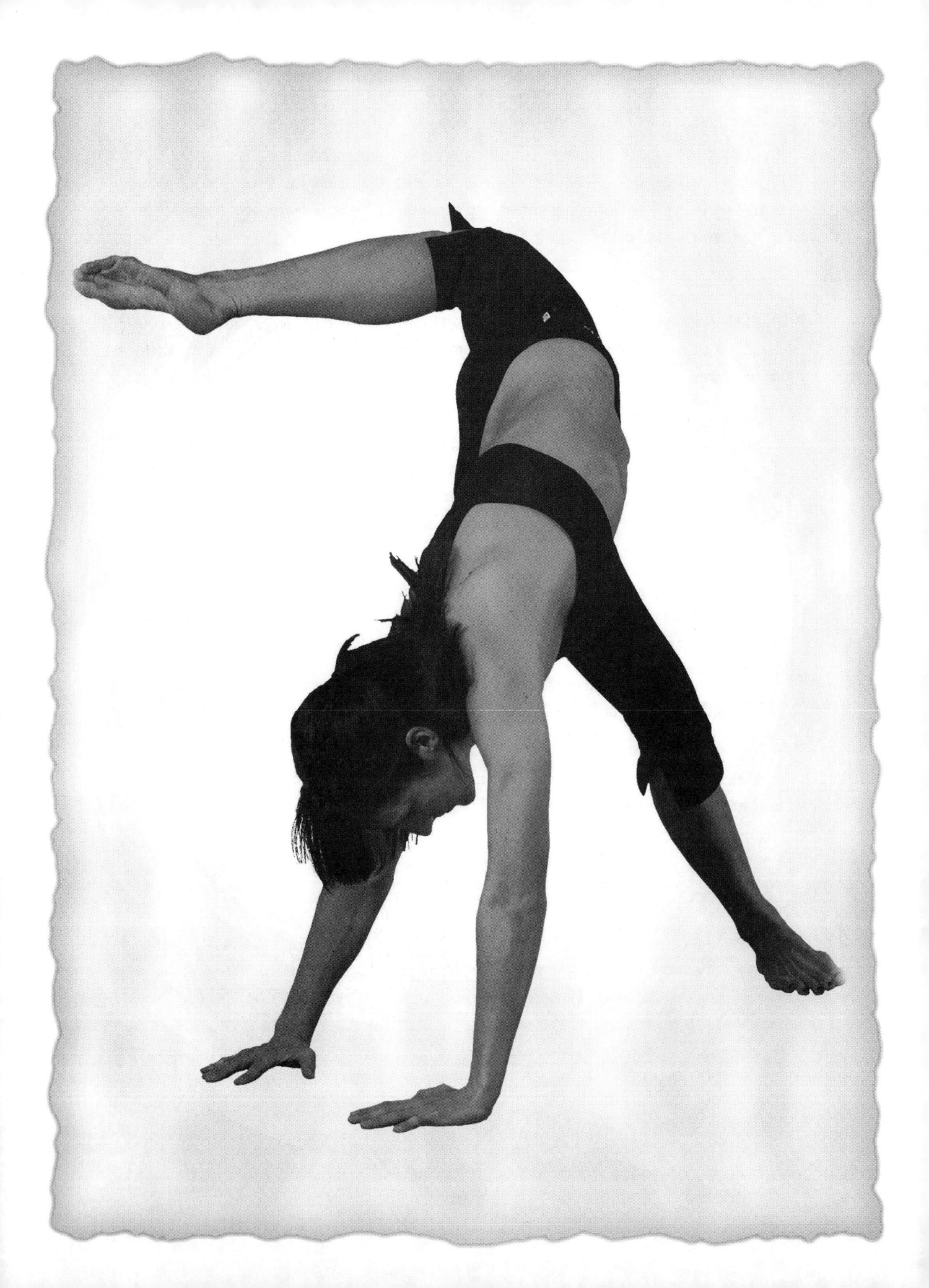

Syncing Breath

How we breathe depends upon what we have stored within our body. We often cannot merely choose our breathing in our yoga. Usually, we discover an issue and it causes us to gasp and hold our breath. Other times we inhale sharply and attempt to push through, grunting with force. To avoid this fear or force takes daily, consistent practice. We need the courage to face the emotional and psychological challenges the act of entering a pose or movement presents. We need the discipline to breathe through that which frightens or frustrates us.

Often we think that we can just adopt a certain breath pattern and master a pose or movement. However, as soon as we encounter something worthwhile, something substantial within us, blocking our energies, binding our flow, the stress causes us to drop to fear- or force-level breathing.

For instance, if we begin with Ustrasana, or Camel Pose, we usually need to begin by actively exhaling on the effort of pushing our hips forward because of the strength challenge it presents and the surrender challenge it demands.

Over time of practice, after residual tension, density, and fear-reactivity release, the pose becomes less challenging. We then find that we can inhale and lift our solar plexus toward the ceiling as the restrictions around our rib cage release and allow our lungs to fully inflate.

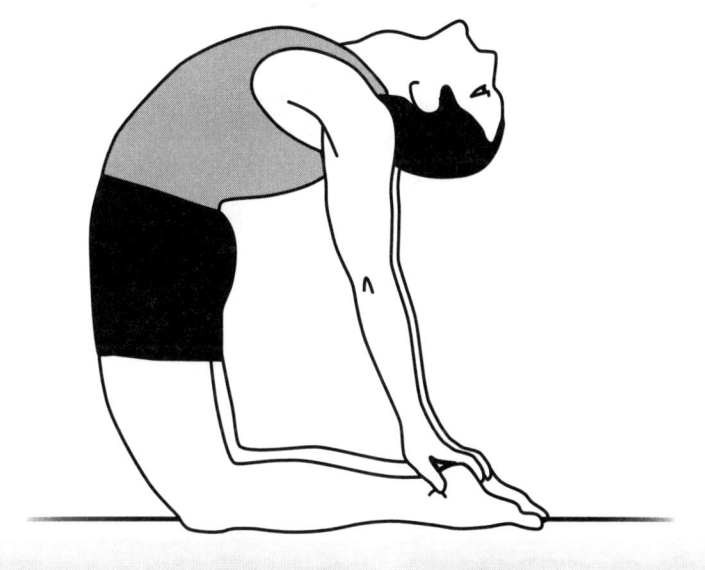

PRASARA YOGA: *Flow Beyond Thought*

The same is true if our strength adapts and progresses to moving through poses. This adaptation and incremental progression process is the central premise of breath mastery through vinyasa. There is a step-by-step process to becoming more masterful in and through all of our poses. The more poses and transitional movement in which we become more masterful, the more transferable that base level of mastery becomes into all of life.

From the following scale, we can gauge our level of mastery in a particular pose or transitional movement by how we breathe.

Breath Mastery Scale

- **Resistance (or fear):** Reflexively inhaling and bracing on perceived effort
- **Force (or anger):** Actively inhaling and pressurizing on perceived effort
- **Discipline (or the beginning of yoga):** Actively exhaling through effort/discomfort; passively inhaling on cessation of effort/discomfort
- **Flow:** Passively exhaling on compression; passively inhaling on expansion
- **Mastery:** The controlled pause after exhalation during the pose or movement

Every time we begin a new pose or movement, if we don't transfer the lessons of mastery to the new learning pose or movement, we need to start at the beginning of the scale again: first fear, then anger, then discipline and, finally, flow and mastery.

Mastery is not only an ongoing deepening process within a pose but also an ongoing expanding process between poses. We must actively work to expand our daily personal practice to include every activity from the time we wake to the time we sleep, in all things: walking, jumping, biking, skipping, talking, driving, writing, typing, tumbling, and so on.

Fear, trauma, and stress — these things can come in and cannibalize our mastery. Mastery isn't a level achieved and neglected. If we're not moving deeper, we're moving backwards. Our breath will always guide us as an insufficient but necessary component of deepening mastery.

Depth of Breath

Breath depth teaches us how to allow the relative intensity of the effort to determine the depth of the breath (as well as to experience the passive inhalation in controlled settings). It relates to three of the four types of breath volume in our lungs:

- **Normal breath:** The volume of our normal exhale/inhale

PRASARA YOGA: *Flow Beyond Thought*

- **Complementary breath:** The volume above our normal breath requiring moderate effort to exhale

- **Supplementary breath:** The volume above our normal breath requiring intense effort to exhale

- **Residual breath:** The volume of breath remaining in our lungs above maximal exhalation

If we're alive, then residual breath is not an issue. We only need to consider normal, complementary, and supplementary breath.

In yoga, these relate directly to skin, muscle, and organ, respectively. The more challenging the pose, the more we must exhale into the challenge. At first, we can only exhale just off the top of our lungs at a clavicular level — the challenge is so great, the fear-reactivity so strong, the myofascial density so thick, the residual tension so tight, the sensory motor amnesia so blind. But over time we relearn the ability to exhale more deeply from the normal breath to the complementary depth into our intercostals. And with protracted practice, we learn to get deeply to a diaphragmatic level through exhaling our supplementary breath depth. With each of the three volumes of air expelled, we become increasingly more stabilized and able to release deeper and deeper bound structures.

Relationship Between Depth and Effort

Force-level breath (aka power breathing) is like injecting foam into a flat tire. It substitutes pressure (compression) for lack of (tensegrity) structure.

Increasing the level of discipline and flow in our breath is like a radial tire, which adjusts air volume automatically appropriate to the needs of the terrain, vehicle, and driver. Its tensegrity is composed of springy steel and proportionate pressure.

At the level of discipline, flow, and mastery, our perceived exertion (RPE) and the depth of breath volume are directly related: As exertion increases, greater volume must be released in order to stabilize the core. In other words, as our exertion increases we move from normal breath volume, to complementary breath volume, to supplementary breath volume at the greatest exertion. In yoga, this allows us to continue to go more deeply into a pose, to first find balance and then apply effort and then to persist.

It is a divine gift to have resistance-level breath to protect us from basic life hazards. It is safer still to have the ability to become angry enough to take action against the imbalances we endure within us. However, with discipline, we can learn to allow flow to erupt spontaneously not just within the pose, and between poses, but throughout our lives.

PRASARA YOGA: Flow Beyond Thought

Skill to Mastery Core Activation Scale

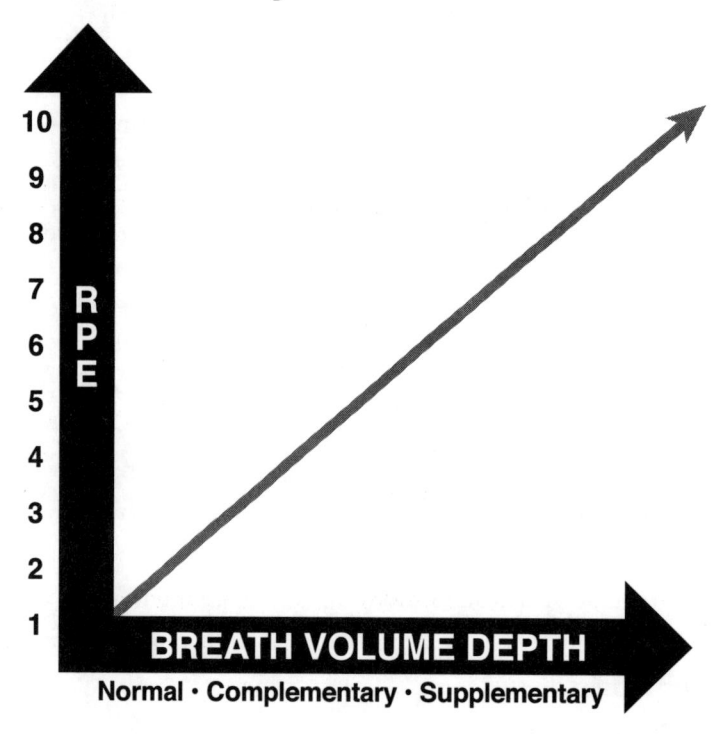

RPE (1–10) vs. BREATH VOLUME DEPTH
Normal · Complementary · Supplementary

Copyright 2005 RMAX.tv Productions

Perpetual Flow

Russian researchers discovered that teaching the segments of a new movement in their sequential order from start to finish is not necessarily as effective as teaching the action in the reverse order (Vorobyev, 1978). They examined the effect of breaking down movements into basic components and having athletes learn each element separately before attempting the whole movement. This method of component learning also proved to be superior to the conventional method of natural sequence learning.

For each yoga flow there is a beginning, middle, and ending component. Once you understand the breakdown process of beginning, middle, and ending elementary motor components, you gain the ability to engineer the educational sequence of movement:

- **Forward engineering:** Learning components from beginning to ending
- **Reverse engineering:** Learning components from ending to beginning
- **Lateral engineering:** Learning middle components, then beginning and ending

These tools work differently for individual learning styles.

One of the crucial secrets to moving from asana to vinyasa and from vinyasa to prasara in your yoga is the movement in between. Every flow has beginning, middle, and ending elementary motor components. Tie together asana into flows. Do this by breaking the asana into elementary motor components.

How is this possible? The goal is to discover that the ending component of one asana flows seamlessly into the beginning component of another asana, forming the chain.

Realize that there is no beginning and ending to movement. Rather, movement in life is composed of only middle components. There is only transition! Realize the movement in between and you gain the ability to analyze any movement as sequences of building blocks and to alter and combine building blocks into any sequences.

PRASARA YOGA: *Flow Beyond Thought*

Every yoga flow involves a beginning, middle, and ending component. Even an asana contains these three components, and in most yoga practices how one enters a pose, the beginning component, is the same as how one departs from a pose, the ending component. In asana, it is the middle component where one concentrates on finding the balance of strength and surrender, and once one does, applying effort, and once one can, applying persistence.

Once we've been able to persist in two asana (most yoga teachers suggest three minutes as a measuring stick), then we can begin to sequence or link them together. We must be able to breathe through the transition between the two asana. In particular, we must be able to discipline the breath (exhale through the effort). If we cannot exhale through the effort of transitioning between the two asana, then we need to concentrate more on the departing asana, the arriving asana, and the transitional asana.

The departing and arriving asana are easy enough for us to understand, but we often find it difficult to wrap our mind around transitional asana because they are sometimes not orthodox positions. We must realize that the purpose of moving to vinyasa is to synchronize our breath with the transition. We have already integrated our breath within the two asana, but now we must breathe between them.

How is this possible? The goal is to discover the ending component of one asana and how it flows seamlessly into the beginning component of another asana, forming an unbroken kinetic chain.

THE SUN SALUTATION EXAMPLE

We have simple examples in the basic Sun Salutation (Surya Namaskar).

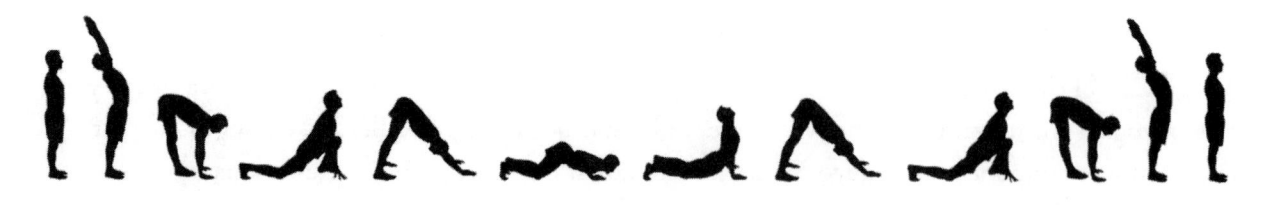

FINDING A MATCH

Each pose flows into the next without transition. Sometimes the end of one pose matches immediately with the beginning of the subsequent one. Other times a component must be added or removed so that they match perfectly. In the first illustration above, Pranamasana, or Mountain Pose, is the beginning and ending component of the second illustration, Hastauttanasana, or Raised-Arm Pose. Salutation Posture is also the beginning component of the third illustration, Padahastasana, or Forward-Folding Posture. Having Raised-Arm Posture match both the ending component of one asana and the beginning component of the

PRASARA YOGA: *Flow Beyond Thought*

next creates a seamless transition, and makes breathing through the vinyasa a simple matter of understanding the breath of the next asana in the sequence. So, actually, the match looks like this transitioning from Salutation Pose to Raised-Arm Pose to Hand-to-Foot Pose (illustrated right):

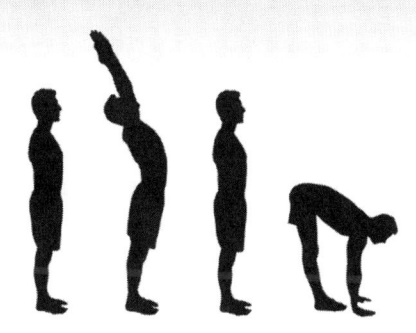

HEMMING IT UP

Sometimes we remove a component in order to transition seamlessly. For instance, the third pose in the Sun Salutation sequence is Padahastasana, or Forward-Folding Posture. Practiced just on its own, the beginning and ending components are the same, as we usually depart from a pose in the same way we enter it. So, if we were practicing Forward-Folding Posture on its own, we would begin with Pranamasana, or Mountain Pose, then move into the Forward Fold to work on the balance of strength and surrender, to apply effort, and to persist. However, in the case of this Sun Salutation we do not depart from the Forward Fold back to Mountain. Instead, we remove that final Mountain Pose component and move right into the beginning component of the next asana, Ashwa Sanchalanasana, or Lunge Pose. By removing the ending component of Forward-Fold Pose, we have seamlessly transitioned into Lunge Pose by squatting and stepping forward with one leg. As a result, this sequence would appear like this:

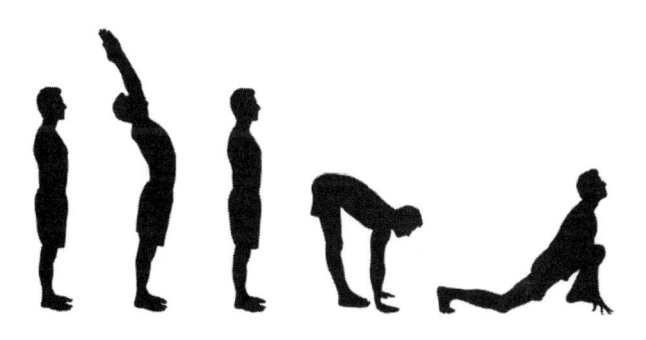

ADDING A PATCH

Sometimes we have to add a component to get to the next pose. In the case of the fifth illustration in the Sun Salutation, Parvatasana, or Downward-Facing Dog Pose, we are intending to move to Bhujangasana, or Upward-Facing Dog Posture. To get there we add the component of moving down like a caterpillar, or Ashtanga Namaskara. As a result, we move from the middle component of Downward-Facing Dog directly into the middle component of Upward-Facing Dog. The example is a little more elegant in that the ending component of Downward-Facing Dog and the beginning component of Upward-Facing Dog have both been removed, as we insert the new component of the Caterpillar. As a result, it looks precisely as depicted in the Sun Salutation sequence above.

PRASARA YOGA: *Flow Beyond Thought*

WE ARE ONLY IN TRANSITION FROM ONE THING TO THE NEXT!

In the cyclical evolution of Hatha yoga, we are never only concentrating on exclusively structure, exclusively breath, or exclusively movement. They are ubiquitously present. We are working to unite them, as in the origin of the word *yoga*.

In asana, we focus on balancing strength and surrender within a pose, implicitly involving breath and movement. In vinyasa, we focus on syncing the breath through and to asana, implicitly involving movement and structure. In prasara, we focus on finding flow between asana, implicitly involving structure and breath.

Prasara, due to the historical evolution of yoga's arrival to American shores, has been a lost method. However, it's inherent in the language already employed within extant teaching methods.

In asana, we must move into and out of a pose in the same way. The movement into the pose is the first component, the movement out of the pose is the final component, and what most people consider the asana itself is the middle component. However, the asana includes this beginning and ending component. Asana implicitly includes prasara. Prasara is only the union of the ending component of one asana with the beginning component of the subsequent asana. Thus, when we embody prasara, we stop *doing* yoga and start *being* yoga.

In vinyasa, we must breathe through and between asana. In asana we learn how to breathe through a pose, but in vinyasa we rediscover how breath guides us to the next movement. By learning to breathe between, we are focusing on moving between, and as a result, we are implicitly involving prasara. By embodying vinyasa, by learning to breathe through events and between them, we stop *doing* yoga and start *being* yoga.

We must realize that there is no beginning and ending to movement. We are only ever in transition from one thing to the next. Life is composed of one endless series of middle components.

The more that we compose flows, the more creativity we express and the more that we unlock our ability to spontaneously respond to any situation with authenticity, integrity, and grace.

Understanding these tools, we can look at all human movement as strings of fluid components. Life returns to being one unending flow. We stop *doing* yoga; we start *being* yoga.

From Recovery to Coordination to Refinement

Our yoga practice evolves along a specific universal path (albeit a cyclical not a linear one):

- **Recovery:** Through asana we release fear-reactivity, discharge residual muscular tension, break up myofascial density, and awaken sensory motor amnesia.

- **Coordination:** Through vinyasa we synchronize our breath into our movement between structures to produce a synergy from our natural capabilities.

- **Refinement:** Through prasara we integrate our movement into our synchronized breath and structure to increase our efficiency — the physiological expression of harmony — and expand that practice into all things.

Yoga is about baby steps from recovery to coordination to refinement. There's no cookie-cutter program for yoga. When we learn anything for the first time, especially a new physical skill requiring our bodies to perform in a certain manner, there are three stages of motor science we go through as biomechanisms.

Psychologist Paul Fitts has described the three stages involved in learning a new skill (Thomas David Kehoe, 1997) as follows:

- **Cognitive:** When we learn the performance goals of the skill, we must consciously regulate and control each skill nuance.

- **Associative:** When we practice the skill, our skill timing and rhythm refine unconsciously, increasing fluidity.

- **Autonomous:** After protracted practice, the skill becomes automatic and unconscious.

In the cognitive phase, we concentrate upon integrating three physical virtues: breathing, movement, and structure. We must pay extreme attention to the detail of the asana nuance.

PRASARA YOGA: *Flow Beyond Thought*

In the associative stage, we no longer need to concentrate on the external performance goals of the skill in order to regulate the movement. Our attention can transform into effort. Effort involves the internal sensation of our skill performance goals. We experience the outcome of each performance goal inside of us, and learn where we must apply strength, and where we can then surrender superfluous tension. In the autonomous stage, we refine the skill to the level of unconscious performance. We can then transform effort into persistence — the ability to sustain the appropriate balance of strength and surrender often referred to as "selective tension."

Once we have developed an asana to the autonomous stage, we can begin to plug it into a sequence with other asana at an autonomous stage, to synchronize the breath through — but more important, between — the two asana.

Prasara is not linear. It is only after the protracted practice of many vinyasa sequences that we begin to allow prasara to happen, though we can begin prasara as early as the beginning. Flow erupts spontaneously on its own, and in degree. We cannot set a schedule. We can only discipline ourselves to deepen and expand our practice daily.

Through prasara, we develop free-flowing practices where we express our integrated breath and structure through movement. And when we encounter a clunky movement, hardened imbalanced structure, or held, forced breath, we downshift to vinyasa to unbind it, or downshift all the way to asana to recover the appropriate balance of strength and surrender.

Developing Proper Form

Proper form then involves the total integration of each unique expression of movement, structure, and breathing illustrated in this Venn diagram:

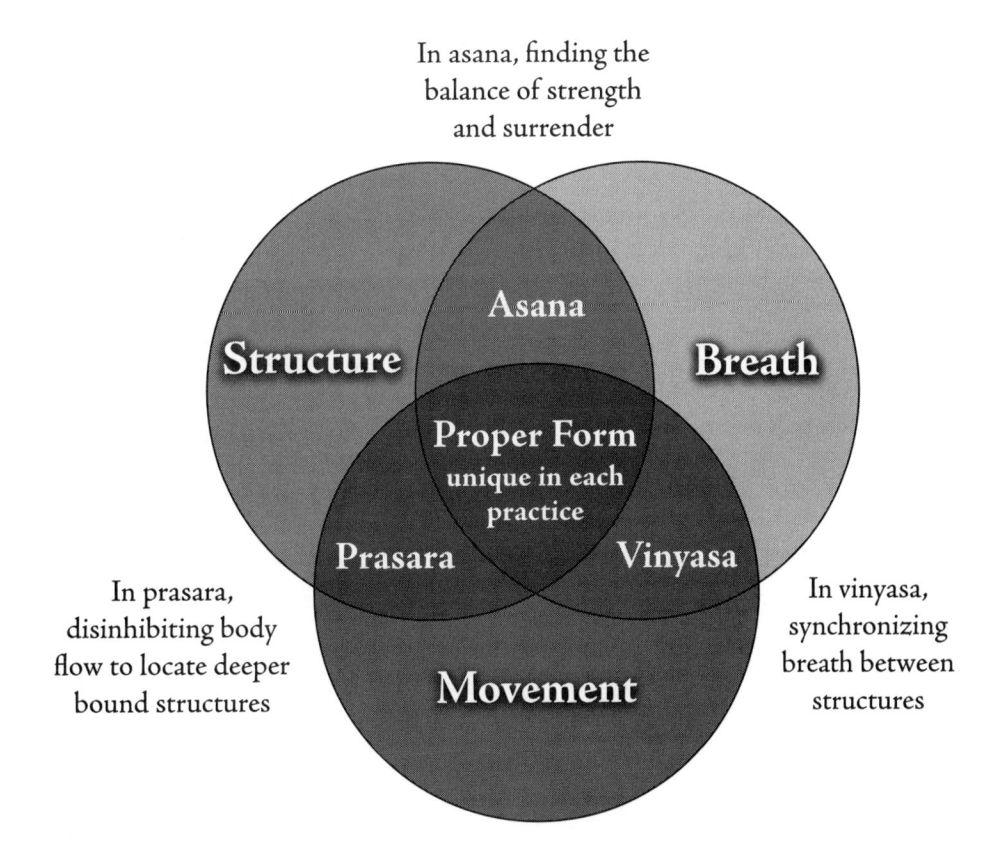

In asana, finding the balance of strength and surrender

Structure — Asana — **Breath**

Proper Form unique in each practice

Prasara — Vinyasa

Movement

In prasara, disinhibiting body flow to locate deeper bound structures

In vinyasa, synchronizing breath between structures

This may appear compartmentalized. However, we of course practice movement and breathing in asana, structure and movement in vinyasa, and breathing and structure in prasara. It is the focus of the method that differs.

PRASARA YOGA: *Flow Beyond Thought*

Our development can be better understood if we extrapolate this two-dimensional Venn diagram into a three-dimensional flower blossom, as it relates to the spiral nature of our personal evolution. We travel around the diagram in constant cycles, moving from asana to vinyasa to prasara then back to asana in smaller and smaller spirals of development toward proper form, not just in our personal practice but in all things throughout our lives.

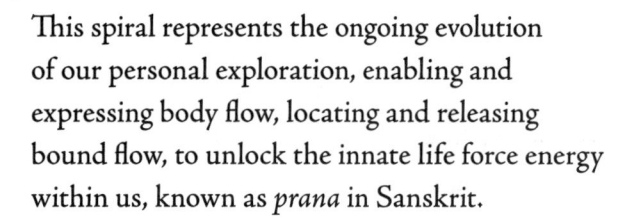

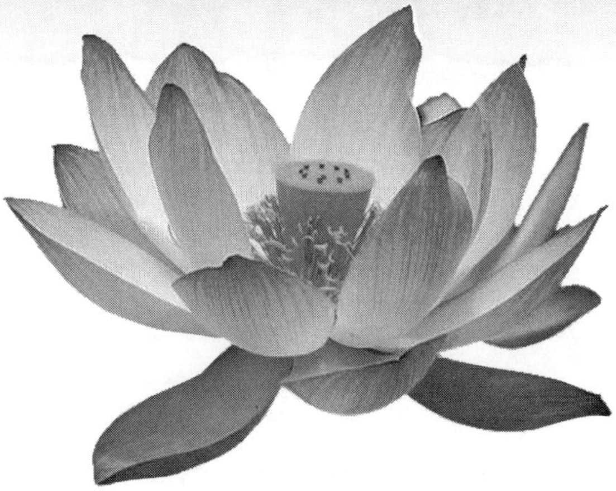

This spiral represents the ongoing evolution of our personal exploration, enabling and expressing body flow, locating and releasing bound flow, to unlock the innate life force energy within us, known as *prana* in Sanskrit.

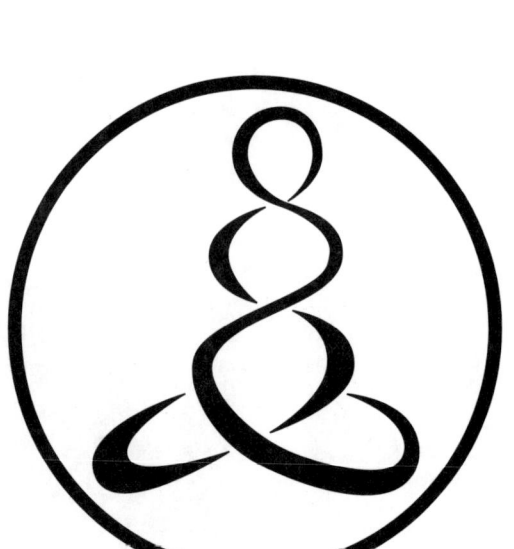

In yoga, the metaphor of the chakras is used to describe how and, to a degree, where bound flow happens. Chakras are a nexus of biophysical energy residing in our body. When we become bound in a particular chakra, that energy becomes stagnant and stifled, manifesting physical issues. When it is released through the practice of yoga, the energy released manifests as body flow. This is a very simplistic description of an elaborate odyssey, which only we as individuals can describe to ourselves, and which the greatest teachers brilliantly illuminate through their questions, practical suggestions, humor, and compassion.

Lotus photo courtesy of PDPhoto.org

Conclusion

This work is intended to convey the natural evolution of yoga through the daily deepening of our personal practice from asana, or balancing surrender and strength in structure, to vinyasa, or syncing breath through and between a series of asana, to prasara, or disinhibiting flow through improvisational exploration and expression of movement.

Certainly, one begins with asana development, the basic education of the alphabet, followed by forming words and sentences through vinyasa development. Then, finally, a conversation erupts spontaneously between you, yourself, and everything. However, this development is not purely sequential, but cyclical.

We begin with asana, and before sequencing them, we develop the ability to balance surrender and strength in a particular structure, intrinsic movement, or field of tension, as well as our breath type, quality, and depth. Once we have to a degree mastered a particular set of asana, we can sequence them in vinyasa.

In vinyasa, when breath disintegrates with the movement between a particular set of asana, we downshift and concentrate on the individual movements in between as new asana themselves. Once we have developed those in-between asana, we resume our vinyasa practice to sync our breath to the sequence. With each new vinyasa sequence we practice, and on any particular day, we will find a multitude of work to do — which will be our yoga for that day.

After serious study of our vinyasa, we have gained the ability to improvisationally explore the union of any connection of points (asana) or string of breath (vinyasa). We can use prasara to converse dialectically with our system to find our yoga for that day. And when we find some hidden point, we can downshift to vinyasa to sync our breath back up with the sequence, or we can downshift all the way to asana to address disintegrated structure if there is an imbalance of surrender and strength.

Prasara is much more than merely an expressive yogic dance. It is much more than merely an exploratory diagnostic tool for identifying covert disintegration of our movement from our breath and structure.

PRASARA YOGA: *Flow Beyond Thought*

Prasara is how we expand our personal practice into everything we do at every moment. By expanding prasara off the mat and into our lives, we plug into where we are and how we are addressing the situation at hand at any particular moment.

Prasara is how we stop *doing* yoga and start *being* yoga.

Om Amriteswaryai Namaha.

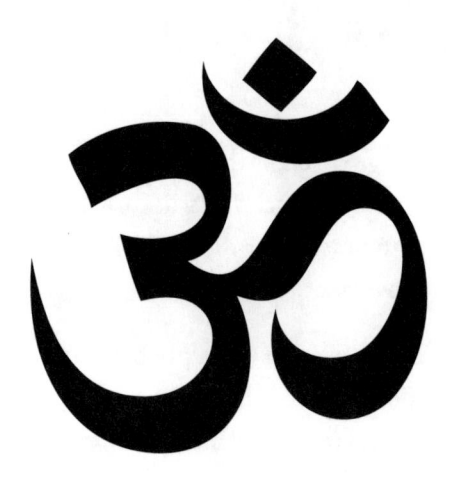

PART TWO

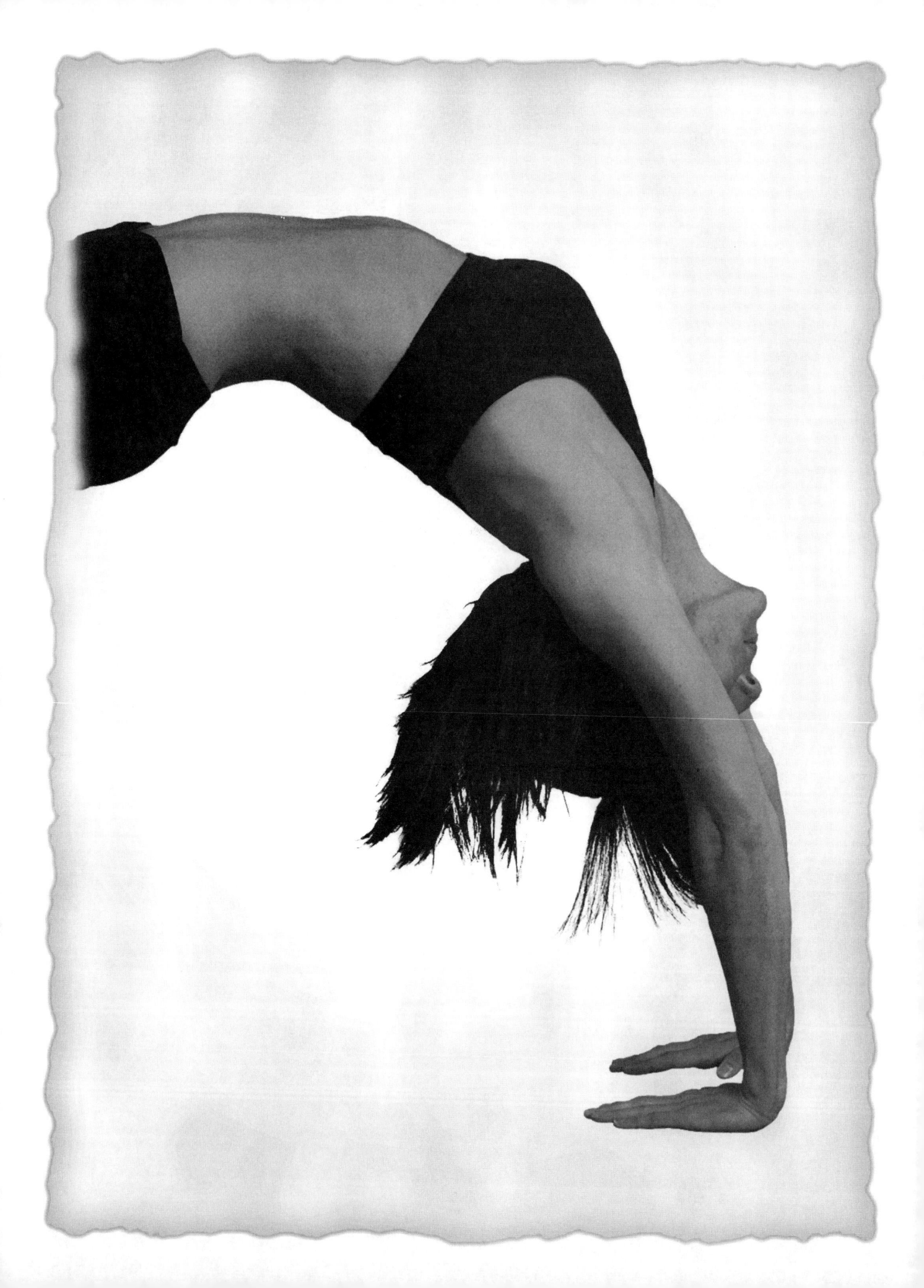

FOREST

PRASARA YOGA: *Flow Beyond Thought*

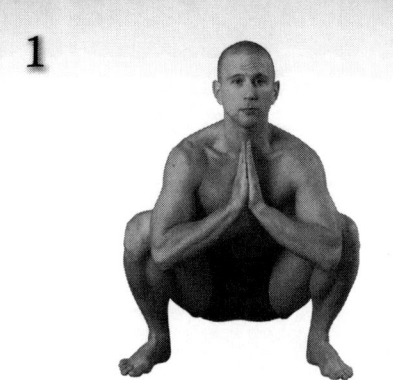

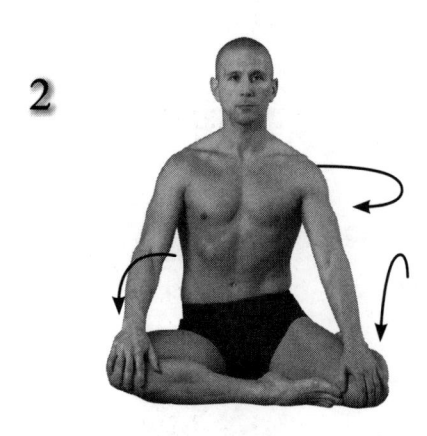

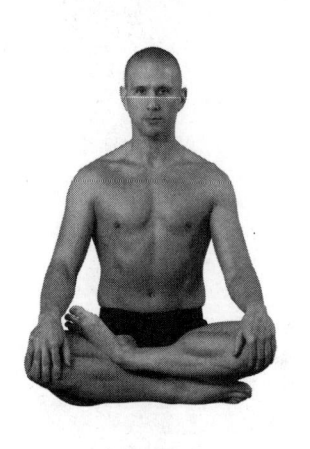

1

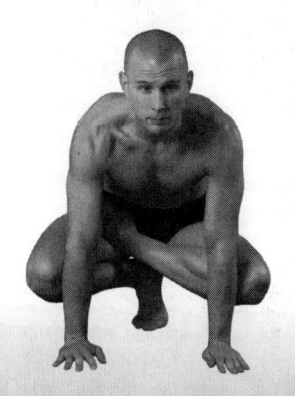

Forest flow begins in standing as you drop smoothly into a Flat Foot Squat (Malasana). Keep your chest tall and crown pulled up as you sink your hips back and down. Exhale as you allow your tailbone to curl under you and drop between your hips (1).

2

Next, you will perform the Shinbox Switch to the right. Allow your right leg to rotate outwards to contact the floor with the outside of your right knee. At the same time, your left leg rotates inward to place the inside of your left knee to the ground in front of your hips (2).

Transition smoothly into the next asana by continuing to turn your body toward your right side. Grasp your left foot with your left hand to bring it over the top of your right thigh (3). This posture is called Fire Log Pose (Agnistambhasana). Your left leg will be nestled deep in the crook of your right hip. Keep both sit bones on the ground in this pose.

3

Now, lean forward and lead with your chest as you place both hands down in front of you, bringing your head toward the ground and folding your upper body over your crossed legs (4). This is Half Lotus Forward Fold (Ardha Baddha Padma Padottanasana). In leaning forward you shift your weight forward and allow yourself room to rise onto the ball of your right foot.

4

PRASARA YOGA: *Flow Beyond Thought*

Flow smoothly into the next position, pressing through your hands and your right foot. Straighten your right knee and walk your hands back, until you are standing tall. You are now in Tree Pose (Vrksasana). Grasp your left foot to lift as high as you can to your edge, but without pain. Press your left knee outward to fully open your hip, keeping your hips square and level. Be long through your upper body to stand tall and proud (5).

Inhale as you bring your left knee up to your chest and grasp just above your left heel with your left hand. Exhale as you extend your left leg and point your toes in front of you (6). This is the Extended Hand Pose (Utthita Hasta Padangusthasana). Once your leg is extended fully, make sure that your hips are in line with each other facing forward. The hip of the outstretched leg should not be further in front than the hip of your supporting leg. Again be firm and stand tall.

Bring your left knee in close to your chest again, and take your left hand over and around your foot to grasp the inside part of your left heel. Exhale as you now lift and extend your foot straight out to the side. You are now in Lateral Leg Lift Pose (Uttihita Pandagusthasana). Bring your right arm out to the side for balance as you keep your hips square and facing forward.

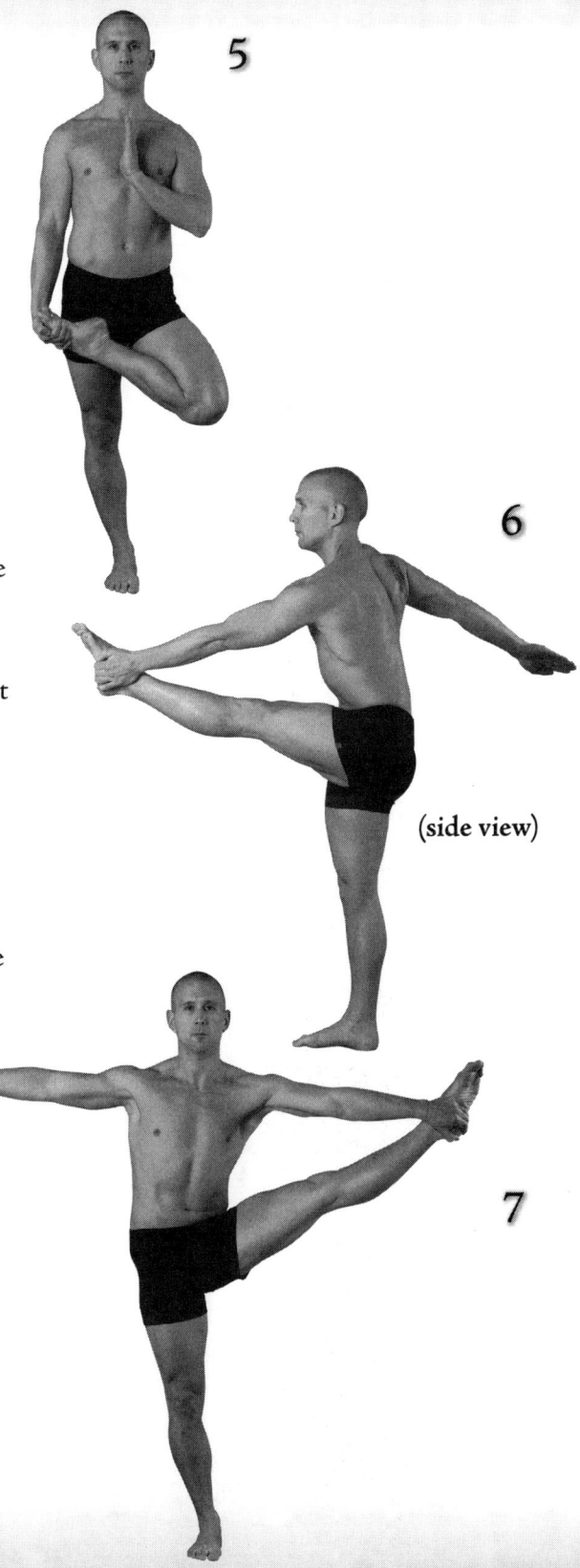

(side view)

III

PRASARA YOGA: *Flow Beyond Thought*

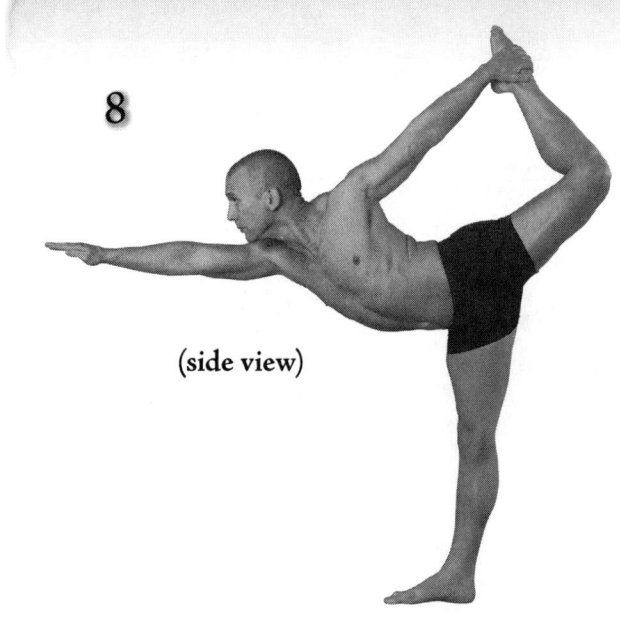

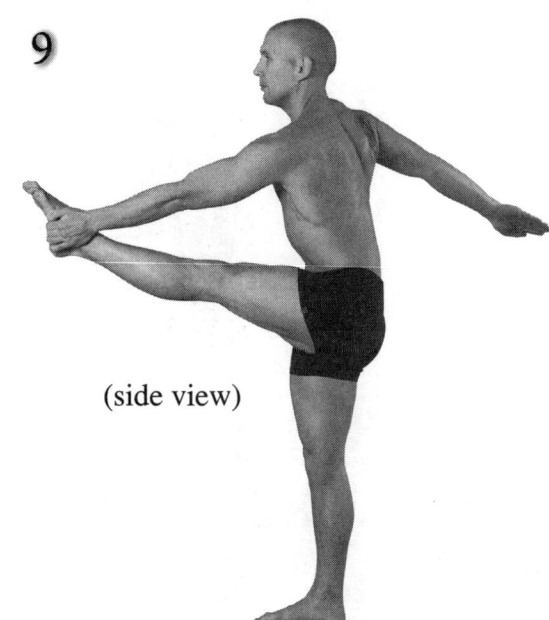

8

(side view)

9

(side view)

Flow smoothly to the next posture by pulling your left knee in toward you. After you pull in tight to your chest, this time bring the knee down to the side of your supporting leg. Your kneecap should be facing the ground as your left hand shifts grasp to the front of your ankle. This is the beginning of Standing Bow Pulling Pose (Dandayamana Dhanurasana).

Bring your right hand up to chest level straight out in front of you. It is very important to keep your hips facing forward in this pose. If you feel your hips turning outward, make a conscious effort to guide them back facing toward the front. Exhaling, pull your left leg up and push your foot against your left hand. This pose is done correctly when you push out against the hand rather than pulling the leg up behind you. As you start the "pull and push" motion, extend your front arm forward and work toward leveling out your back leg with your forward arm (8).

Move out of the position gracefully by bending your left knee and pulling it in toward your chest one last time. Extend straight in front of you to engage in another Extended Hand Pose (9).

PRASARA YOGA: *Flow Beyond Thought*

From this position, bring your foot in toward you and bring your right hand around the bottom and outside of your left foot while your left hand switches to the outside of the left heel. Exhale as you grasp your foot to pull in to touch your forehead (10). This is Standing Pigeon Pose (Eka Pada Rajakapotasana). Hold this position and allow your left hip to open as you keep your right leg firm and strong.

Move out of this posture and bring your foot over to the crease of your right hip to finish in Tree Pose. Lean forward smoothly to place your hands on the ground in front of you while maintaining a straight right leg (11).

Bend your knee when your hands are stable on the ground and drop your hips down. You will flow quickly out of the Half Lotus Forward Fold (12) and finish in Fire Log Pose (13).

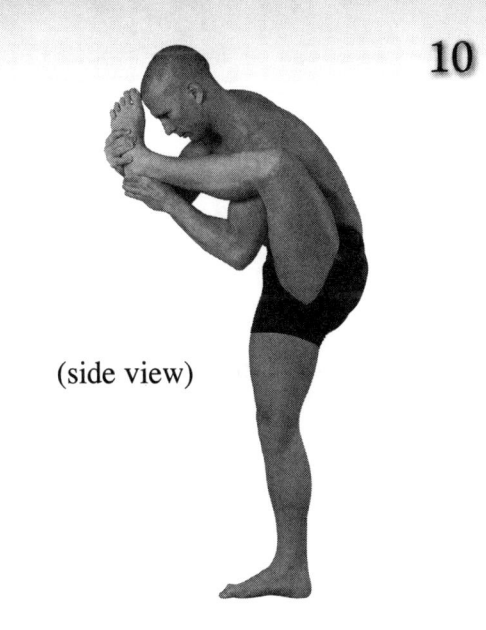

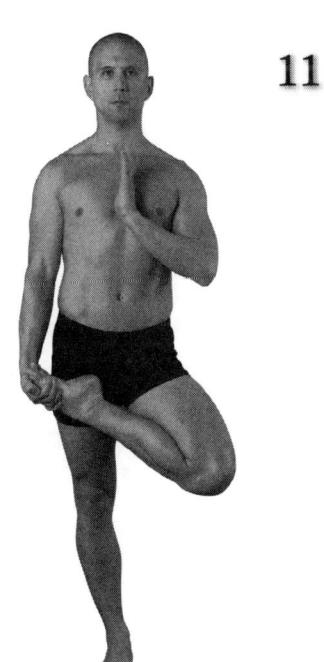

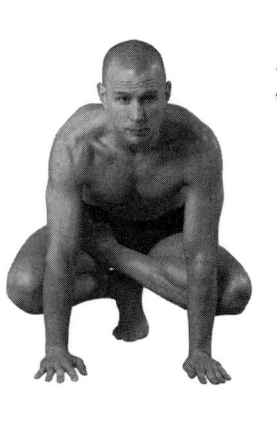

(side view)

PRASARA YOGA: *Flow Beyond Thought*

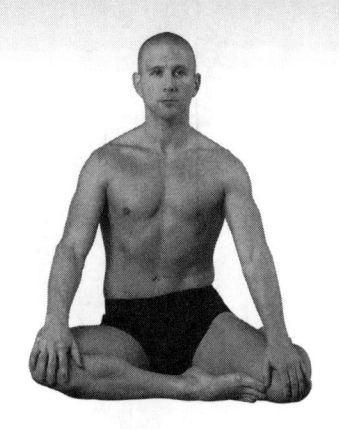

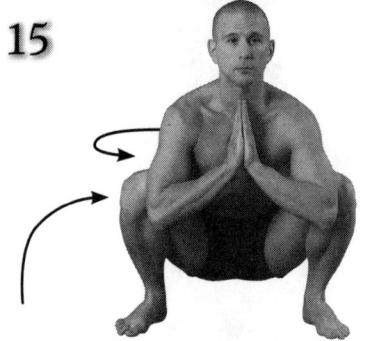

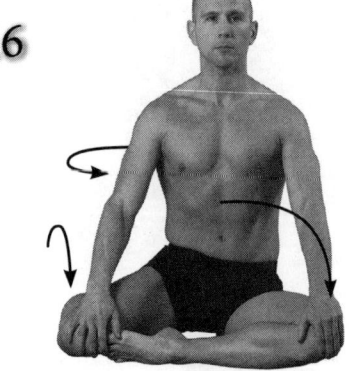

14

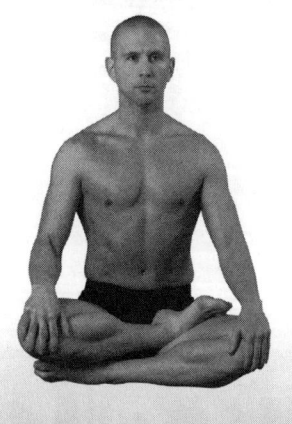

Grasp your left foot and swing it behind you to engage in the Shinbox Position, with your left heel next to your left hip and your right leg folded in front of your hips (14).

Perform a Shinbox Switch (15) to engage in the opposite Shinbox Position with your left leg folded in front of you and your right heel next to your right hip (16).

Bring your right foot up and around on top of your left leg to engage in another Fire Log Pose (17).

Lean forward, placing both hands in front of you for Half Lotus Forward Fold. As in the first half of this flow, shift your weight forward and come up on the ball of your left foot (18).

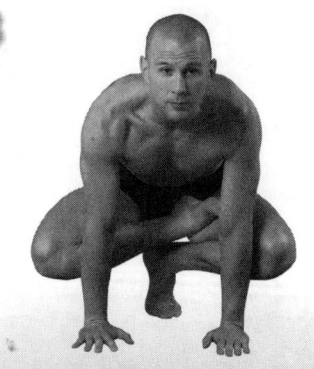

15

16

17

18

114

PRASARA YOGA: *Flow Beyond Thought*

Press firmly through your hands as you straighten your left leg and bring your hips backward. Lift your upper body up smoothly to finish in Tree Pose, with your right leg in the fold of your left hip (19).

You will now engage in Extended Hand Pose, to Lateral Leg Lift Pose, to Standing Bow Pulling Pose, to Extended Hand Pose, and finally to Standing Pigeon Pose (20–24). In this second half of the Forest flow, your right leg is moving through the asana.

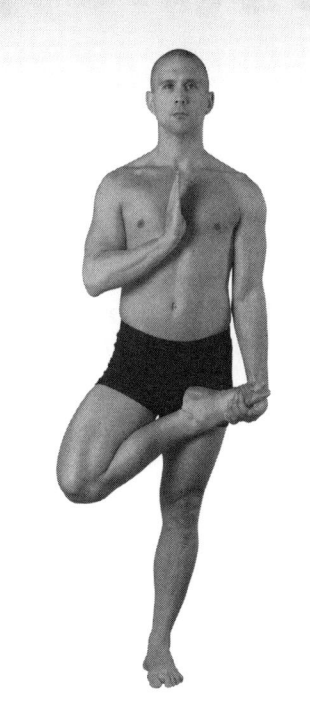

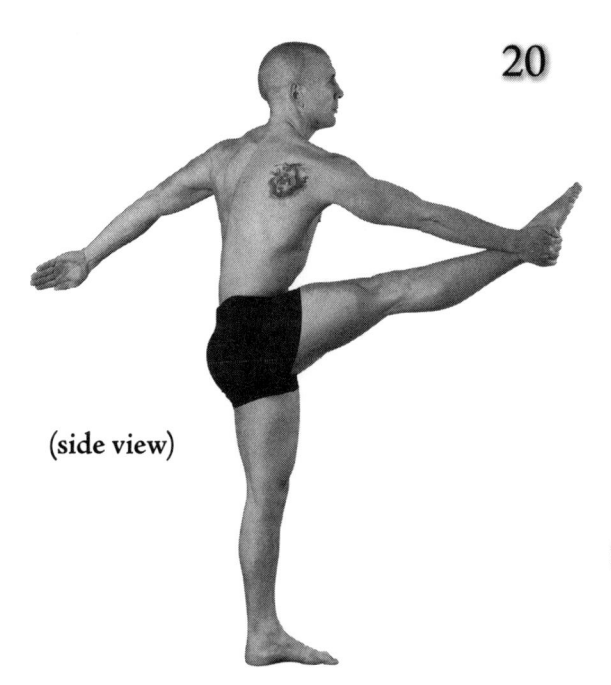

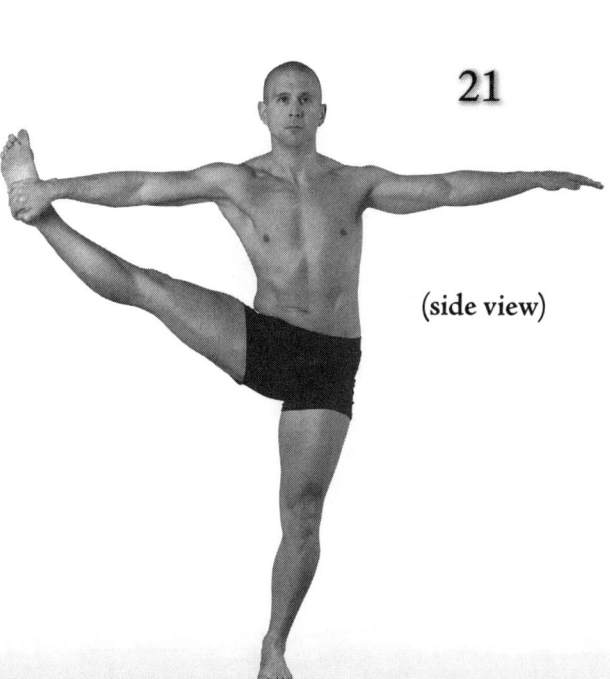

19

20

(side view)

21

(side view)

115

PRASARA YOGA: *Flow Beyond Thought*

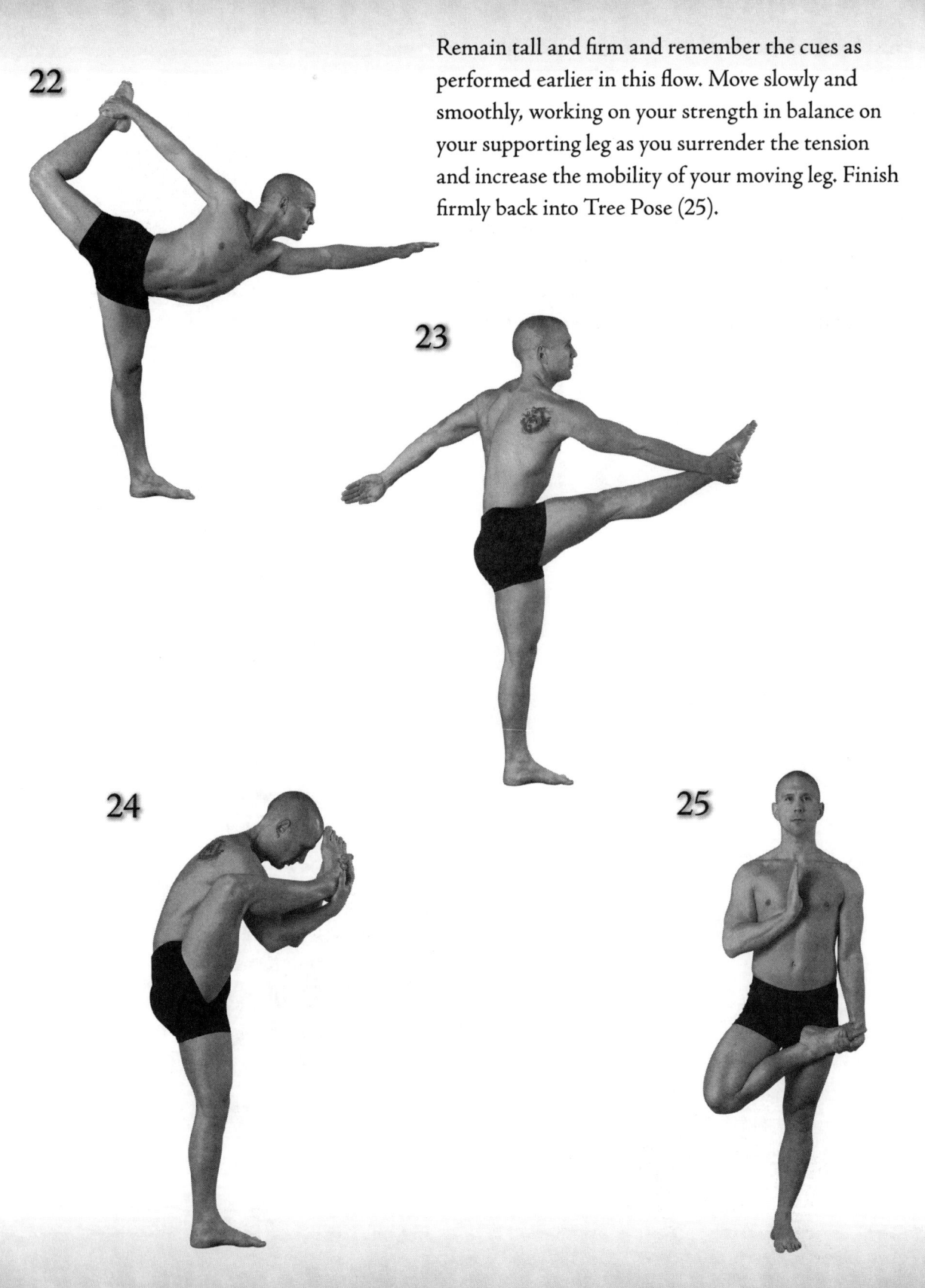

Remain tall and firm and remember the cues as performed earlier in this flow. Move slowly and smoothly, working on your strength in balance on your supporting leg as you surrender the tension and increase the mobility of your moving leg. Finish firmly back into Tree Pose (25).

PRASARA YOGA: *Flow Beyond Thought*

Now lead with your chest and place your hands down in front of you. When firmly rooted, bend your knee and flow smoothly out of Half Lotus Forward Fold (26) to turn to the left and into Fire Log Pose (27).

Grasp your right foot and swing it out and around to the ground to engage in Shinbox (28). Perform the first half of the Shinbox Switch to finish in Flat Foot Squat (29). Rise up smoothly to stand for the conclusion of Forest.

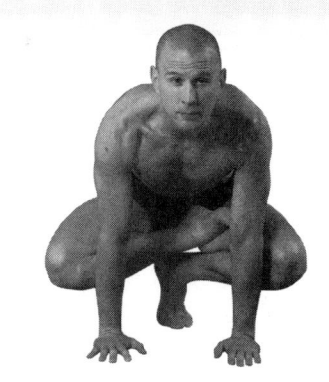

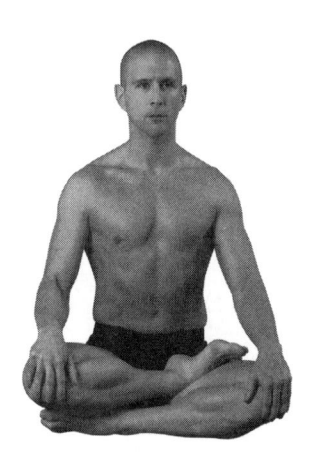

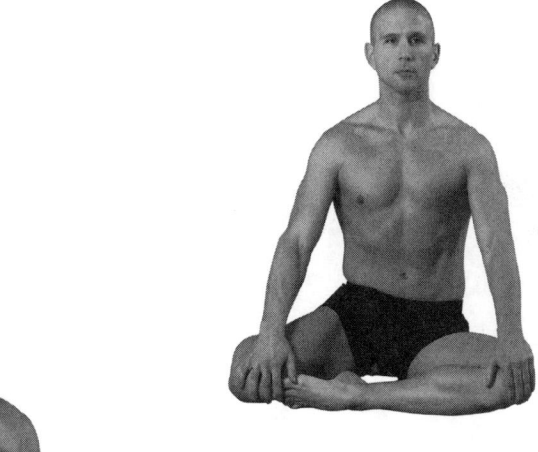

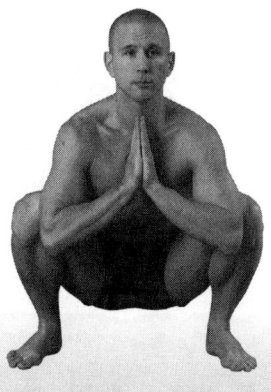

26

27

28

29

117

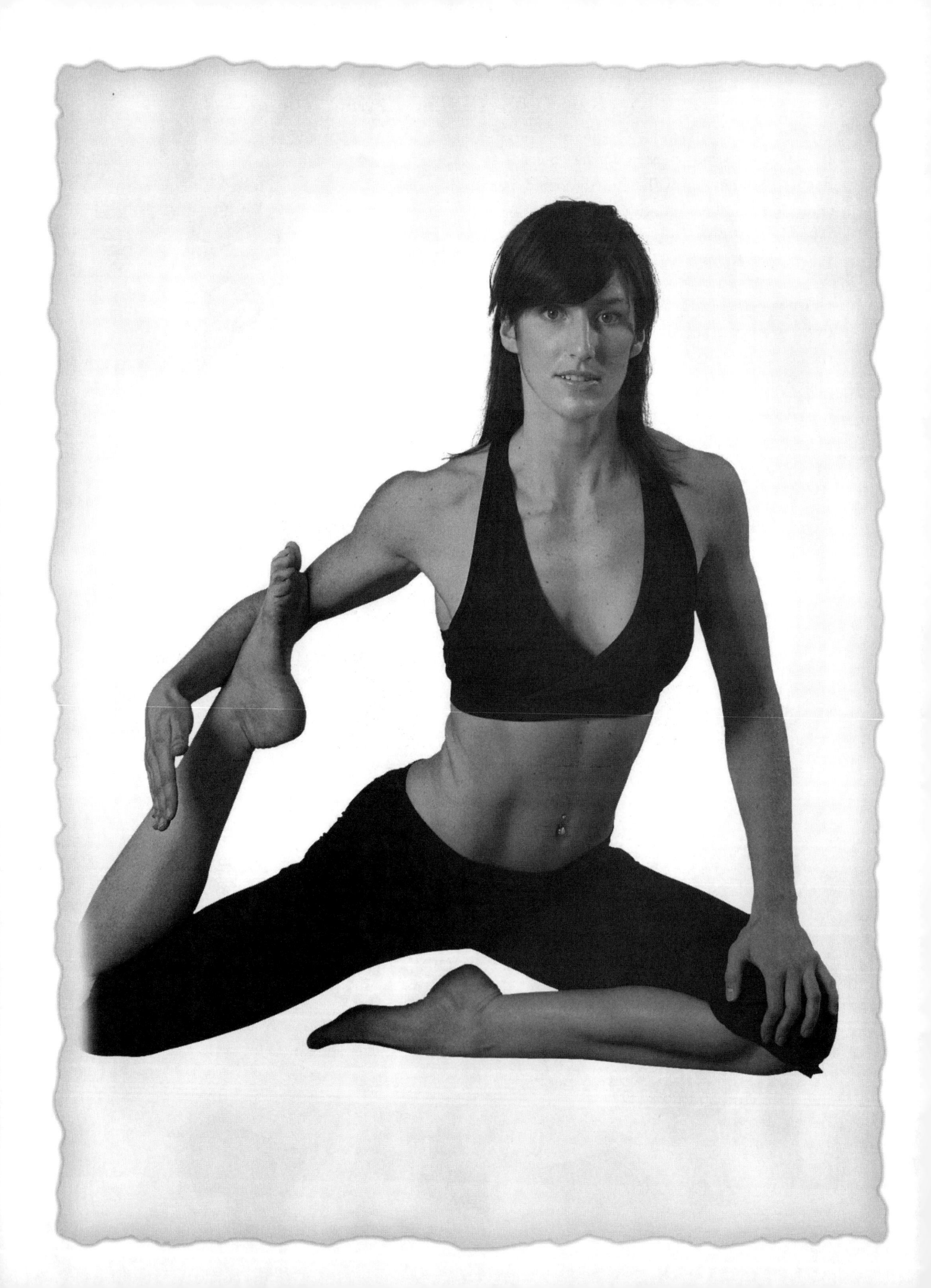

SPIDER MONKEY

PRASARA YOGA: *Flow Beyond Thought*

1

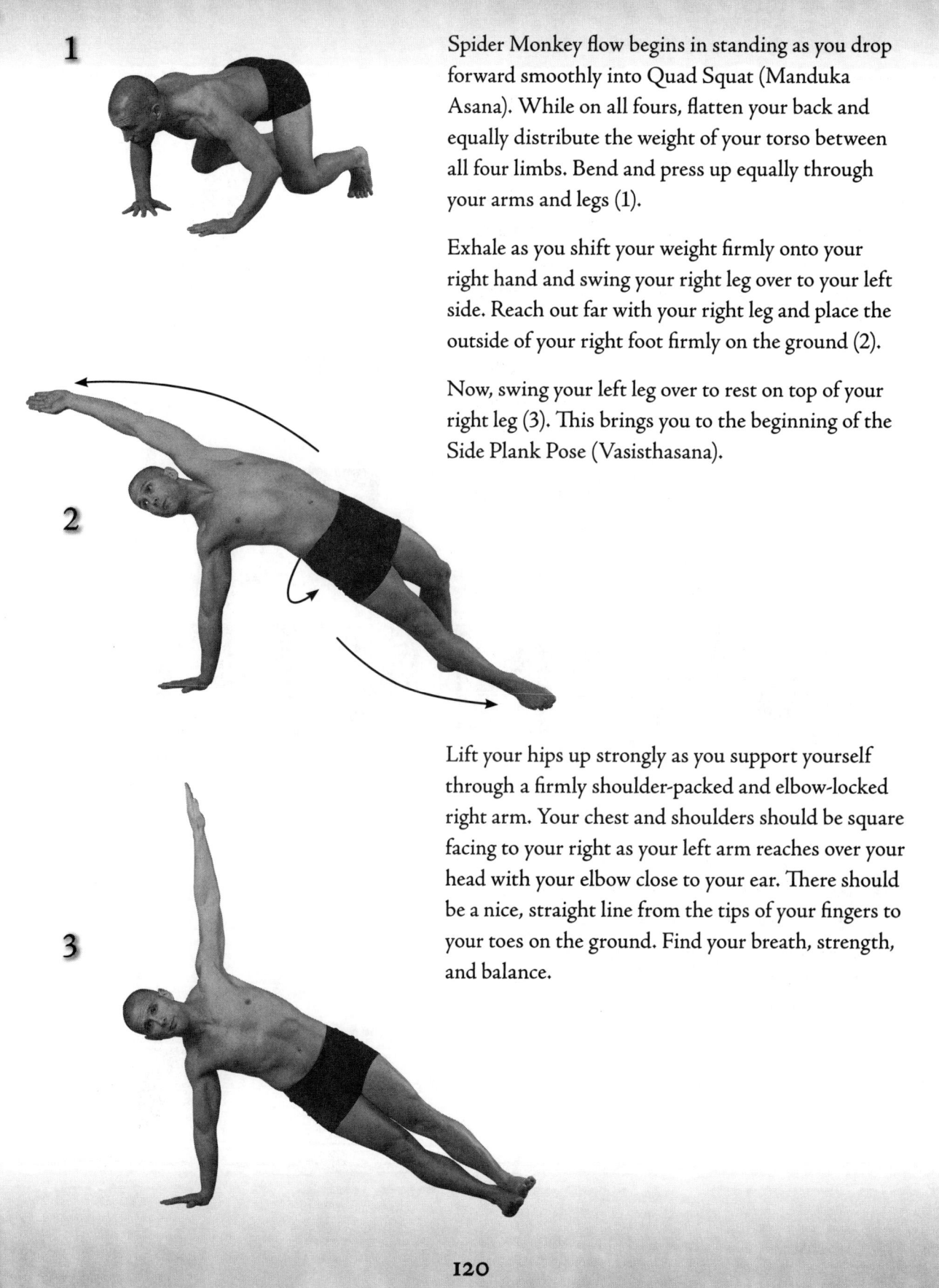

Spider Monkey flow begins in standing as you drop forward smoothly into Quad Squat (Manduka Asana). While on all fours, flatten your back and equally distribute the weight of your torso between all four limbs. Bend and press up equally through your arms and legs (1).

Exhale as you shift your weight firmly onto your right hand and swing your right leg over to your left side. Reach out far with your right leg and place the outside of your right foot firmly on the ground (2).

Now, swing your left leg over to rest on top of your right leg (3). This brings you to the beginning of the Side Plank Pose (Vasisthasana).

2

3

Lift your hips up strongly as you support yourself through a firmly shoulder-packed and elbow-locked right arm. Your chest and shoulders should be square facing to your right as your left arm reaches over your head with your elbow close to your ear. There should be a nice, straight line from the tips of your fingers to your toes on the ground. Find your breath, strength, and balance.

PRASARA YOGA: *Flow Beyond Thought*

Now, lift your left leg high in the air and bring your left hand down to the ground (4). This position is called One Leg Downward-Facing Dog (Eka Pada Adho Mukha Svanasana). This pose is similar to Downward-Facing Dog, except now you will have one leg extended off the ground and raised behind you. Be sure to keep your back flat and do not allow yourself to twist. Keep your hips facing straight toward the ground. Your raised leg and your back should be in a nice, straight line.

From One Leg Downward-Facing Dog, you will perform an Elevated Scorpion (5). In the Elevated Scorpion, you lead with your left knee as you bring it to the sky as high as you are able and reach the knee behind you and to your right side. Keep both hands firmly against the ground as you continue in this twist. Eventually, you will reach the end range of your twist and the motion will bring your left hand off of the ground. Support yourself strongly on your right hand and right foot. Your right leg will bend as your left foot comes to the ground. Exhale strongly as you lift your chest and ribs up high to the sky. Reach your left hand up over and past your head to engage the ground.

You are now in Wheel Pose (Urdhva Dhanurasana) (6). Push firmly through both hands and feet to drive your hips and chest further upwards, elevating in a nice spinal curve. Keep your head in good alignment with your spine while maintaining equal pressure between your hands and feet. The feet should be flat on the ground throughout this pose.

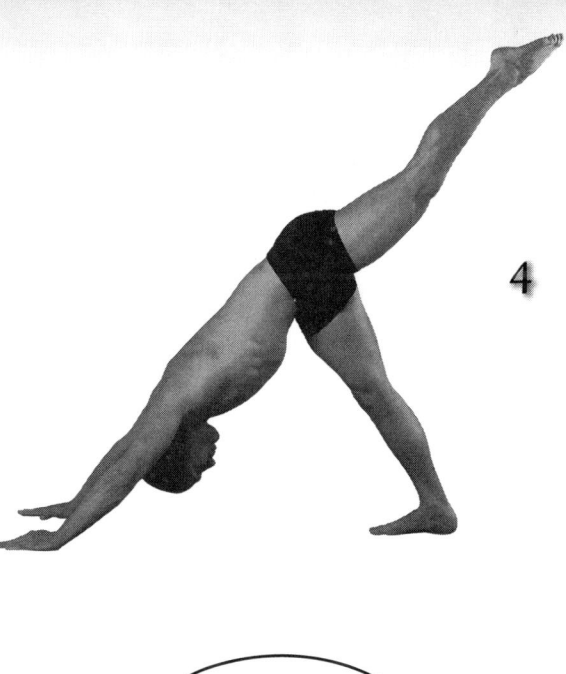

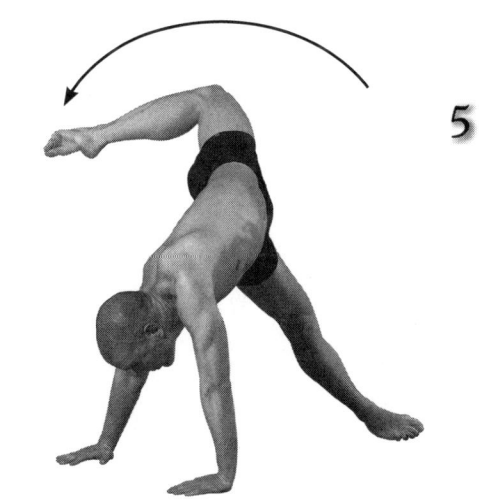

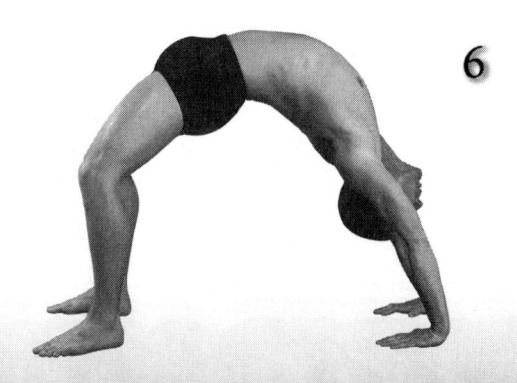

121

PRASARA YOGA: *Flow Beyond Thought*

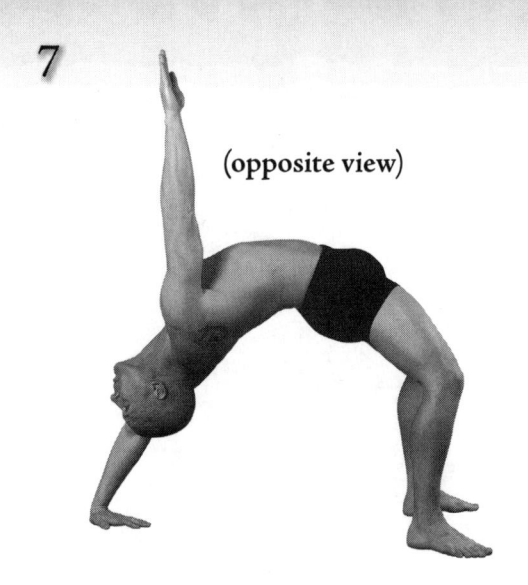

7

(opposite view)

Inhale and keep your chest high to prepare for the next transition. Exhale as you bear more weight through your left hand in order to lift your right hand up off the ground.

Allow your left palm to twist on the ground as you reach over to your left side with your right arm. At the same time, you will bring your left foot back to thread under your right leg. This is called a Threading Bridge (8). You will finish the transition in Quad Squat Position (9).

Now, reverse the process and swing your right leg under you to your left side as you bring the front of your hips up toward the sky. Place your feet firmly on the ground as you reach up and past your head with your left hand (10).

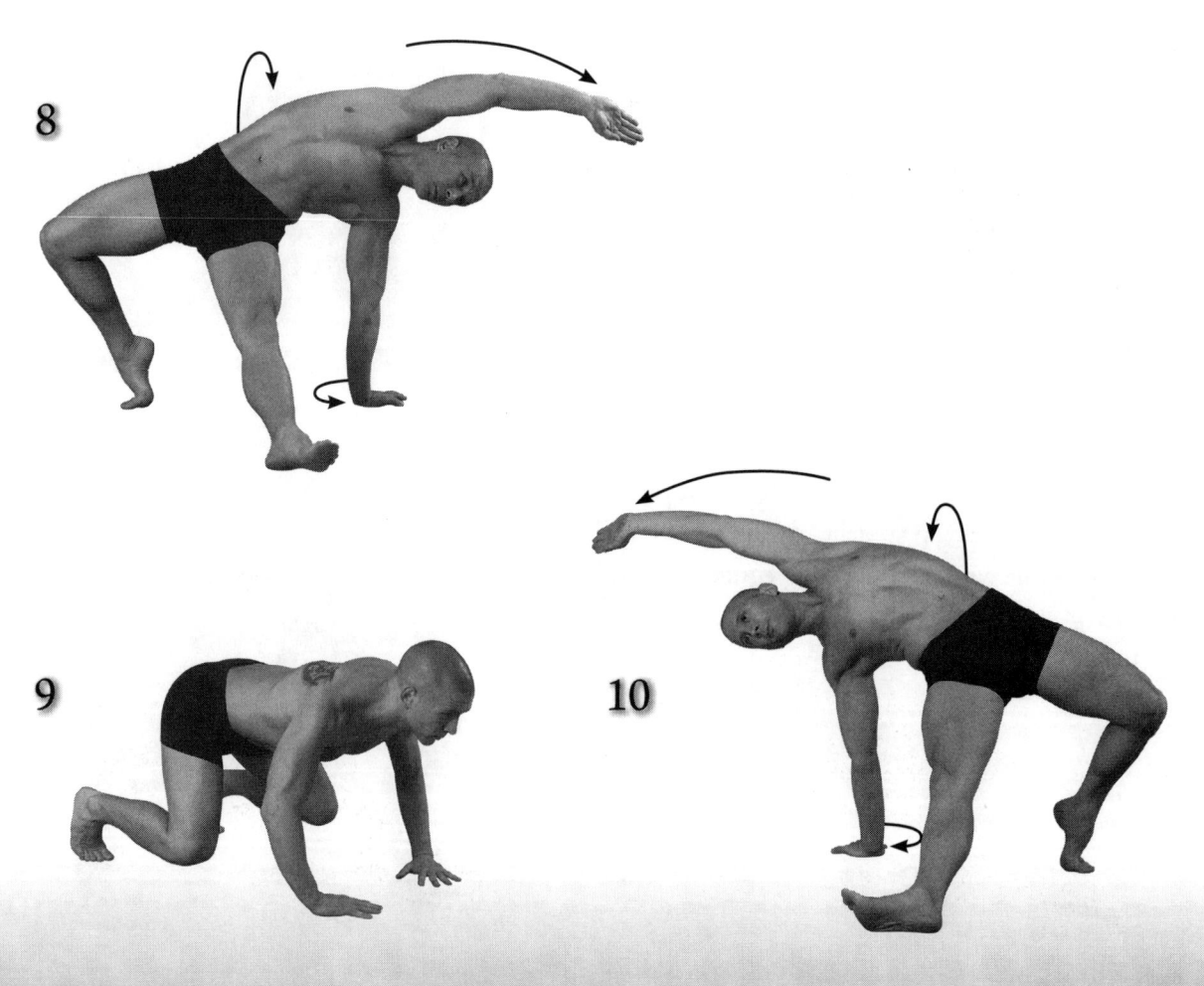

8

9

10

PRASARA YOGA: *Flow Beyond Thought*

Exhale fully, lift your chest and ribs up high, and place your left hand on the ground to engage in Wheel Pose (11). Be firm and strong in this posture, then perform another Threading Bridge (12–13) and bring your right hand up and over to another Quad Squat (14).

You will now engage in Side Plank to the opposite side. You are shifting your weight onto your left hand and now swinging your left foot far to your right side (15).

As described earlier, finish strong and balanced in Side Plank Pose, this time with your right arm up in the air (16).

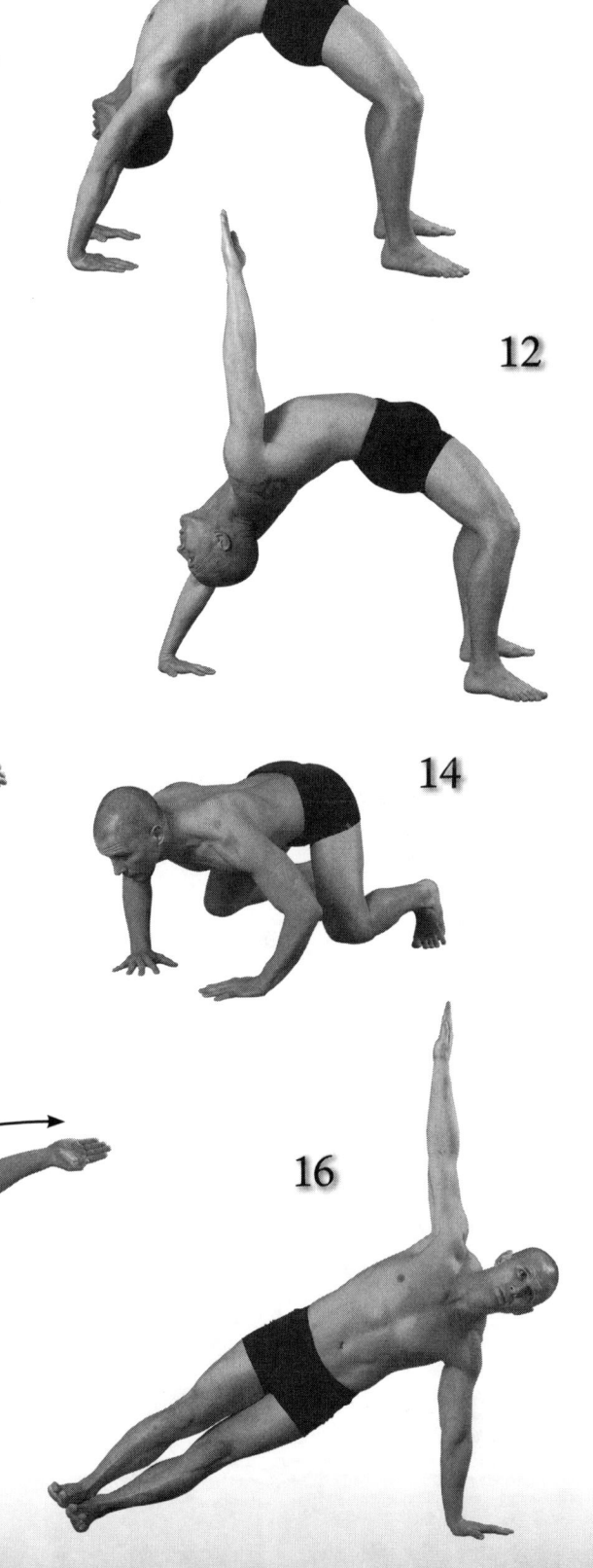

123

PRASARA YOGA: *Flow Beyond Thought*

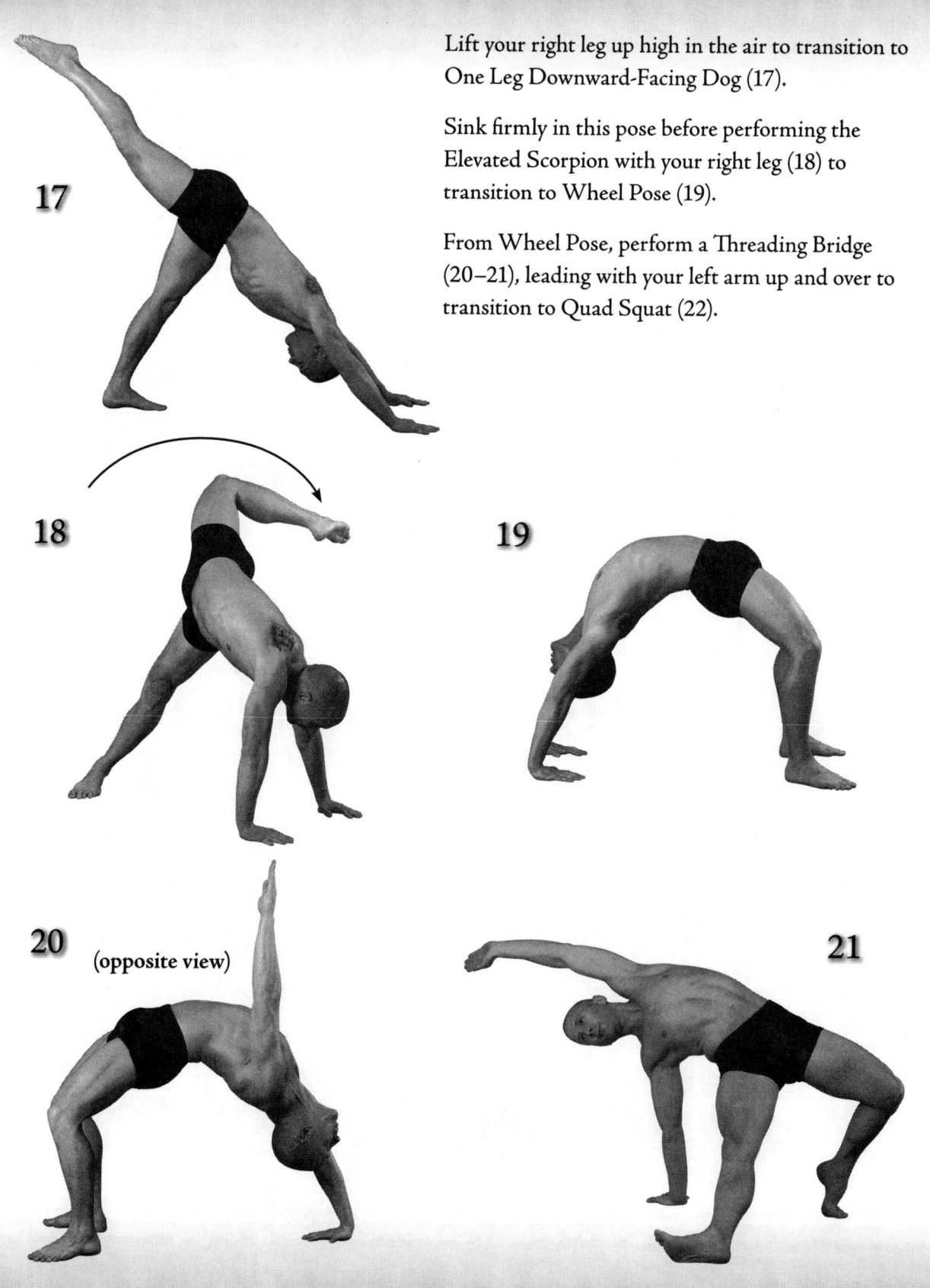

Lift your right leg up high in the air to transition to One Leg Downward-Facing Dog (17).

Sink firmly in this pose before performing the Elevated Scorpion with your right leg (18) to transition to Wheel Pose (19).

From Wheel Pose, perform a Threading Bridge (20–21), leading with your left arm up and over to transition to Quad Squat (22).

17

18

19

20 (opposite view)

21

124

PRASARA YOGA: *Flow Beyond Thought*

From Quad Squat, perform a Threading Bridge, leading with your left leg to flow smoothly into a final Wheel Pose (23–24).

Your last Threading Bridge (25–26) has you turning to your right as your left arm comes up and over to finish in a Quad Squat (27).

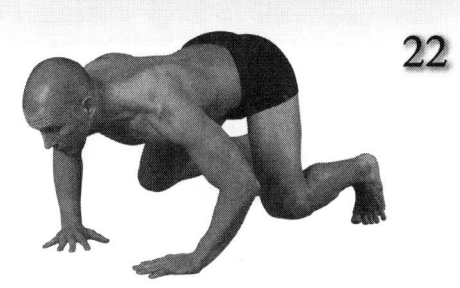

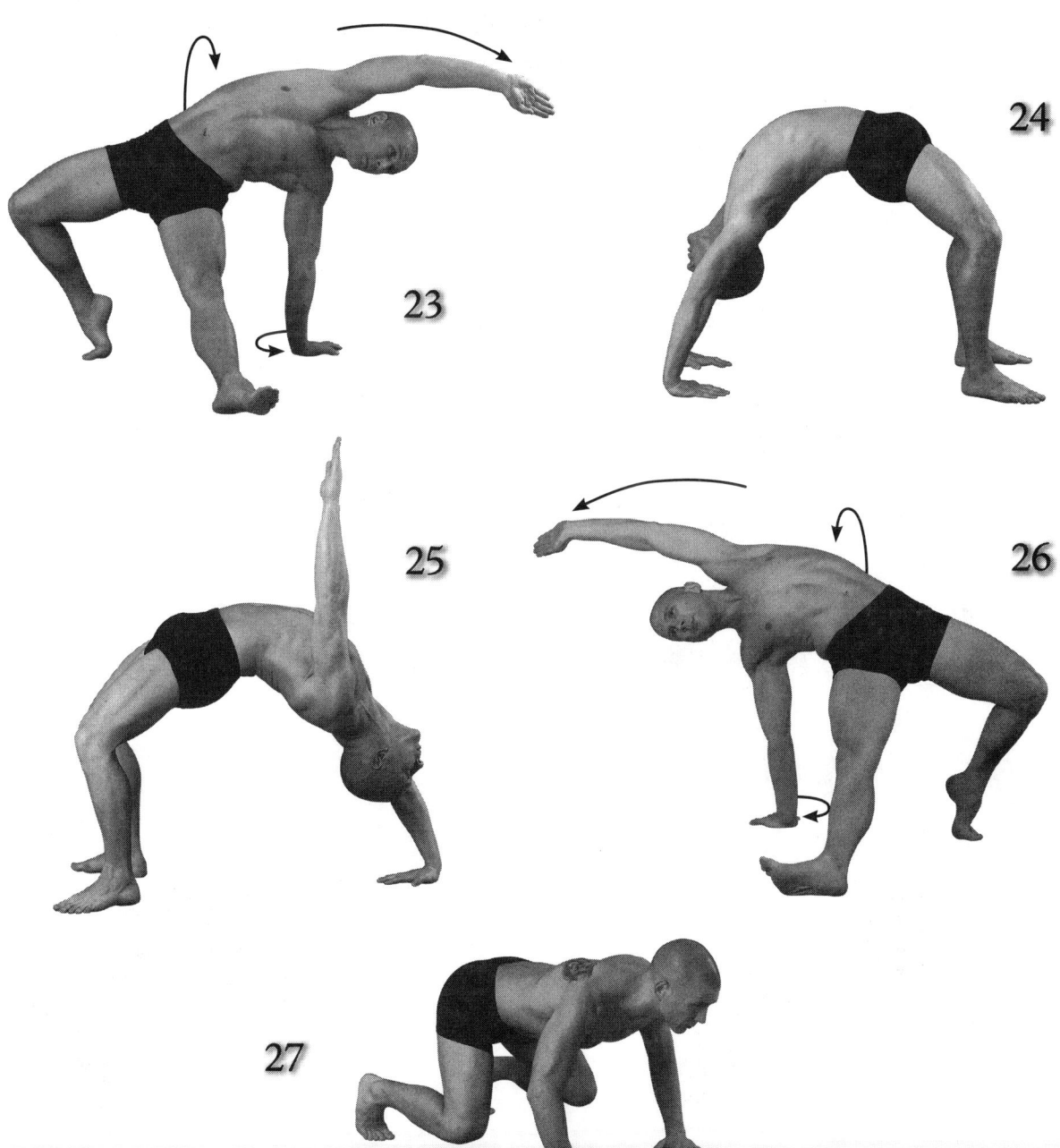

125

PRASARA YOGA: *Flow Beyond Thought*

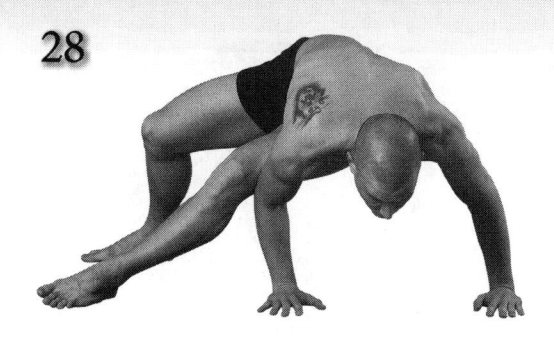

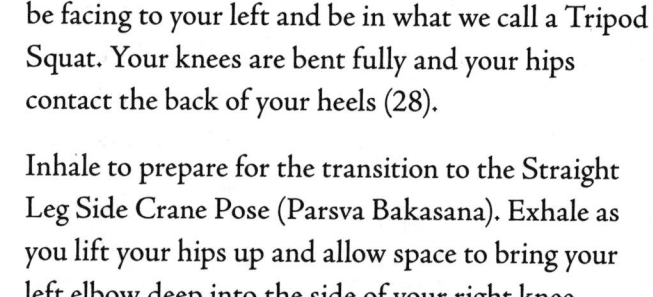

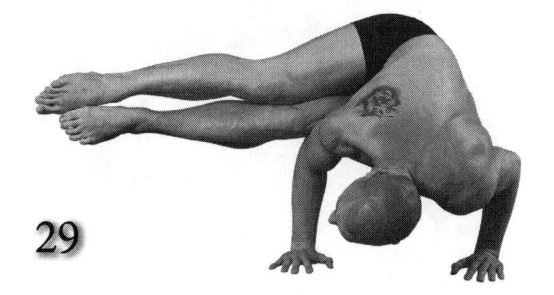

28

Remain in Quad Squat for just a second, and then shift your weight onto your right hand as you bring your right foot to the side of your left foot. You will be facing to your left and be in what we call a Tripod Squat. Your knees are bent fully and your hips contact the back of your heels (28).

29

Inhale to prepare for the transition to the Straight Leg Side Crane Pose (Parsva Bakasana). Exhale as you lift your hips up and allow space to bring your left elbow deep into the side of your right knee. The back of your left upper arm should be resting firmly into the pit of your right knee. Shift your hips to the right and allow your weight to be borne firmly through both arms. Straighten both knees out to finish in a strong, balanced pose (29). Your core should be activated fully and your shoulders are packed and strong. Bring your feet down to transition smoothly back to a Tripod Squat (30).

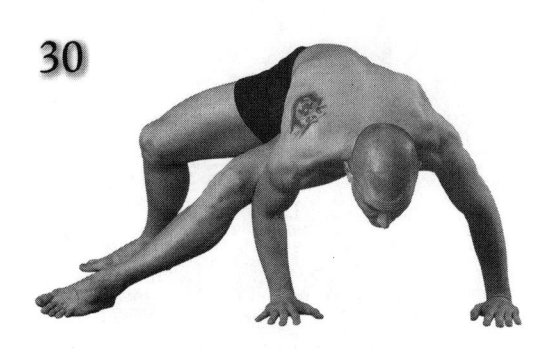

30

From that Tripod Squat you will move deliberately back to a Quad Squat (31); however, do not pause here, simply continue the movement and engage in the opposite Tripod Squat supported by your left arm (32).

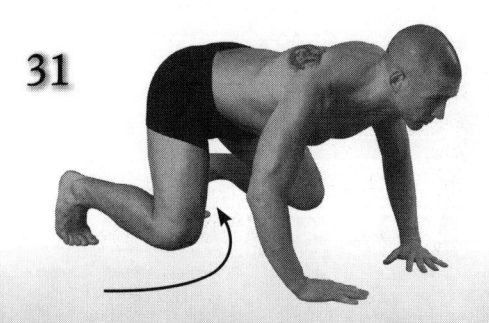

31

126

PRASARA YOGA: *Flow Beyond Thought*

Now you will engage in the Straight Leg Side Crane Pose toward the right side (33). Remember to bring your right elbow fully past the side of your left knee and have your right upper arm firmly in the left knee pit. This is essential to create the stable platform on which to place your legs. Exhale firmly as you shift your hips to the left and end in a nice hand balance.

When ready, flow smoothly out of the Side Crane and back to Quad Squat (34–35) to conclude the Spider Monkey flow.

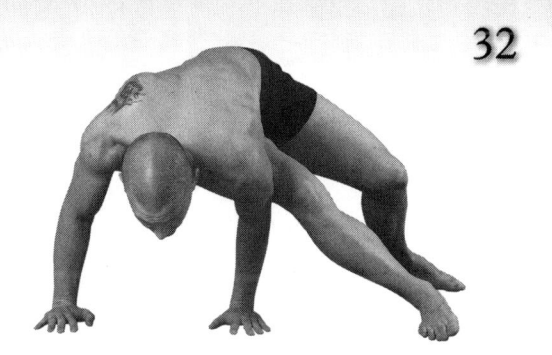

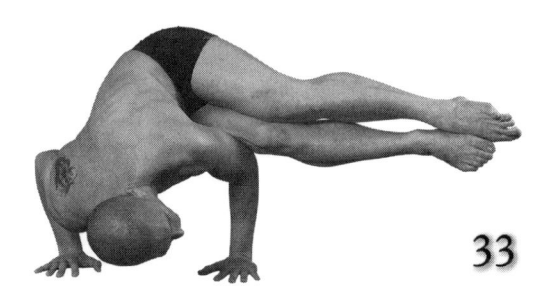

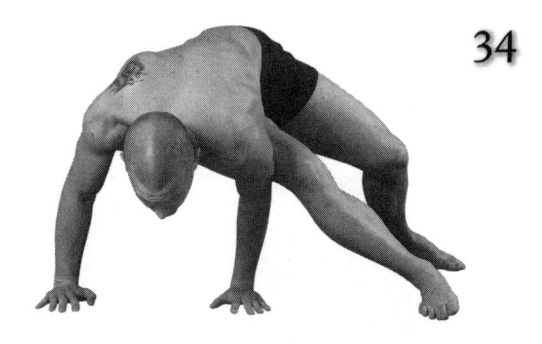

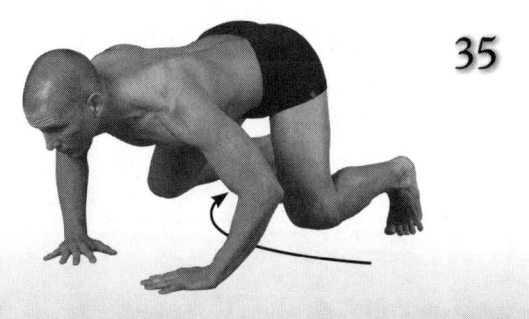

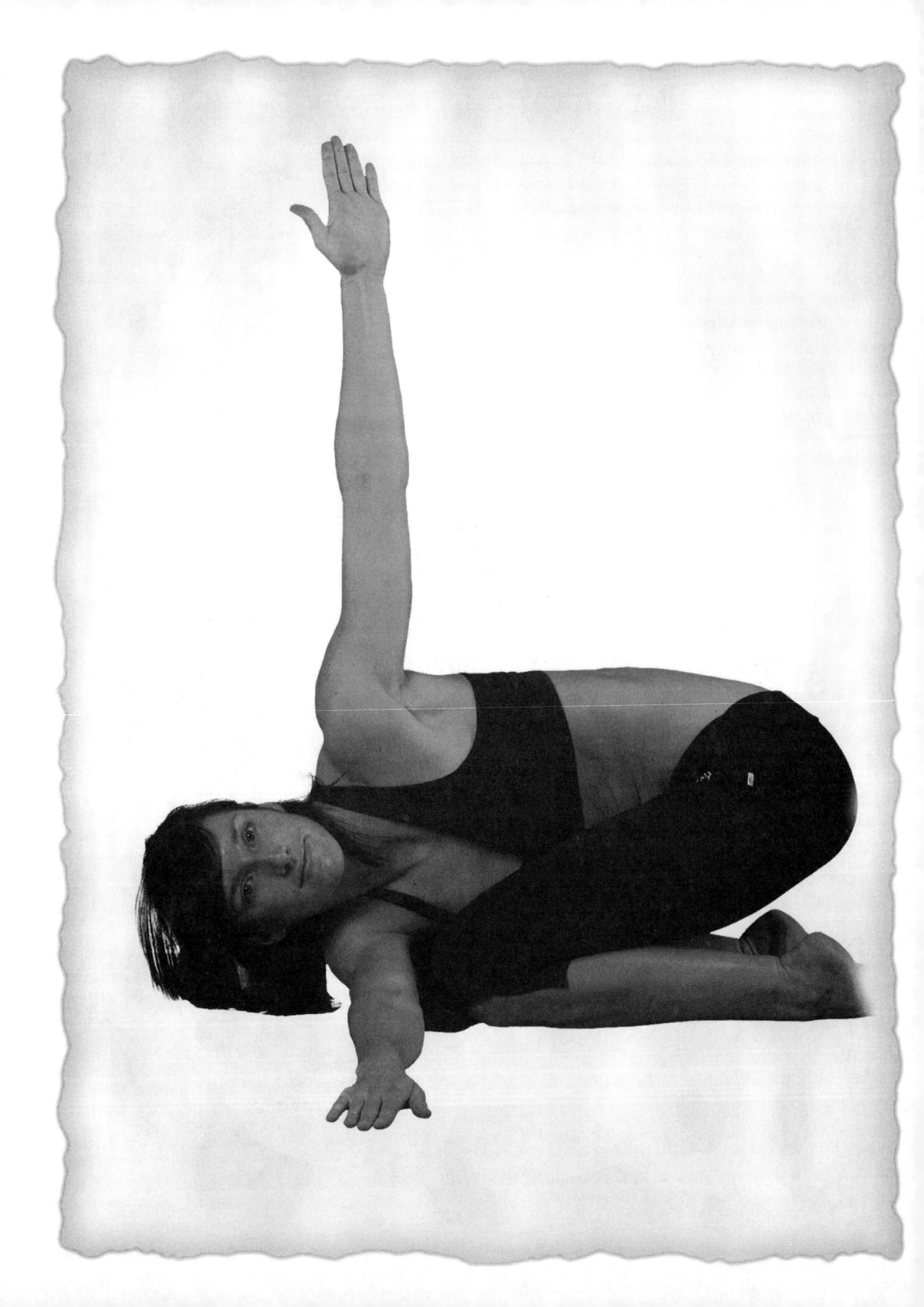

DIVING DOLPHIN

PRASARA YOGA: *Flow Beyond Thought*

1

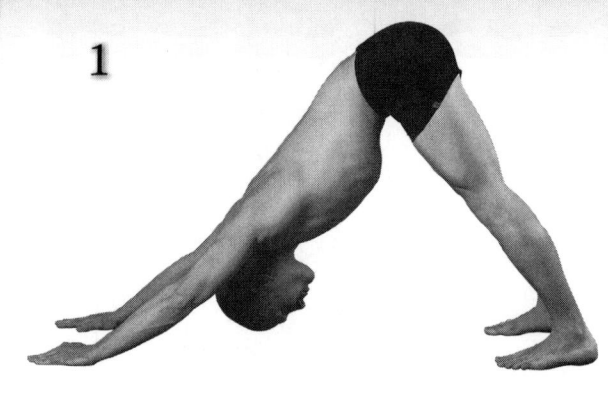

We start the Diving Dolphin flow in Downward-Facing Dog (Adho Mukha Svanasana). Begin on all fours with your hands placed a fair distance from your feet. Keep your hands planted and push with your hands. Your elbows will now straighten to support your upper body as you push your heels down toward the ground. Think again of a long spine and bring your chest downwards toward the floor. Push your buttocks toward the sky and keep your head neutral while looking straight down at the floor. Exhale to sink your structure fully into the asana (1).

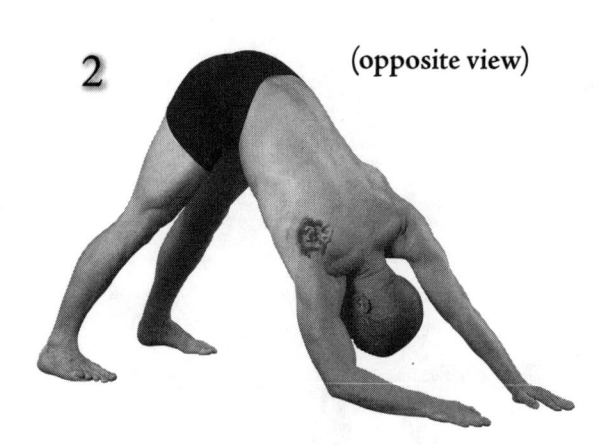

2 (opposite view)

Inhale fully then exhale as you place your right forearm flat on the ground (2). Maintain your crown-to-coccyx alignment and don't allow your spine to twist. Allow your sides to open fully in this movement.

Inhale as you return to Downward-Facing Dog and exhale as you place your left forearm down to balance on the other side (3). Inhale and return to Downward-Facing Dog (4).

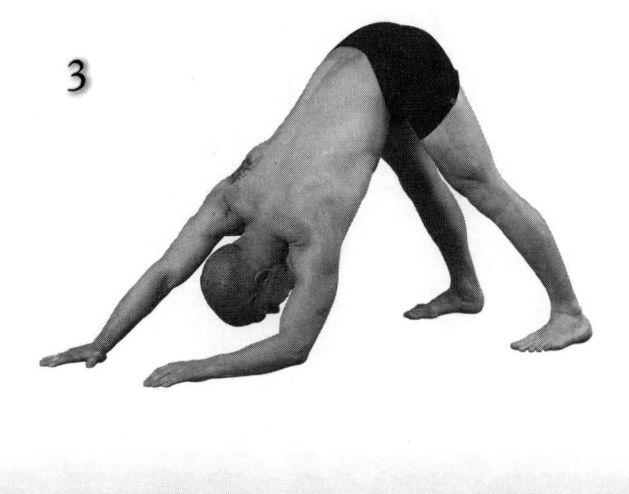

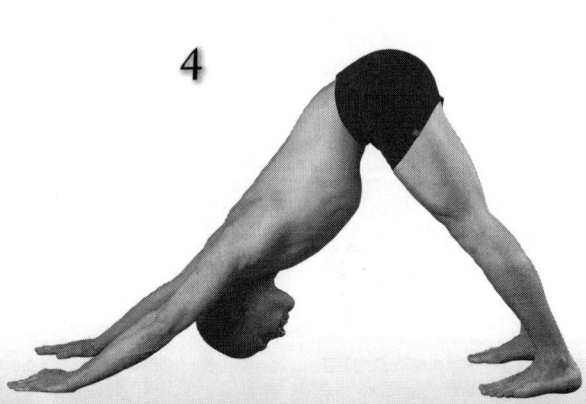

3

4

PRASARA YOGA: *Flow Beyond Thought*

As you exhale to place both forearms down, you are now engaged in the Dolphin Pose (Ardha Sirasana). The mechanics of the pose are as in Downward-Facing Dog, but now you are bearing weight through your forearms instead of your palms (5). Exhale and deepen the pose to your edge.

You will now start a Lateral Roll by dropping your right shoulder to engage the ground (6). Exhale and bring your chin toward your chest to allow yourself to roll onto the back of your upper shoulders. You should not be rolling on your head! As you do this, allow your legs to follow in line with your torso and you will end in the Plow (Halasana).

Rather than trying to touch your toes to the floor, focus on keeping your legs straight and lifting your hips up toward the sky. It helps to think of pushing your chest out and away. This will keep you in proper alignment. Exhale fully as you relax your neck and throat to deepen into the pose (7).

To move out of the pose, you will complete the second half of the Lateral Roll and drop onto your left shoulder (8).

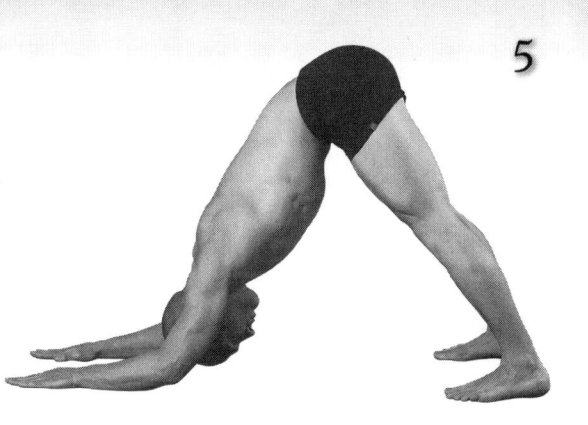

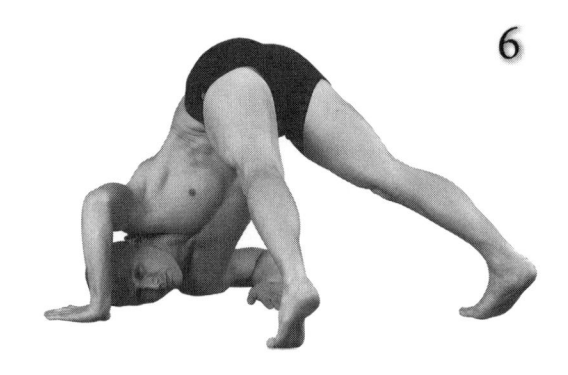

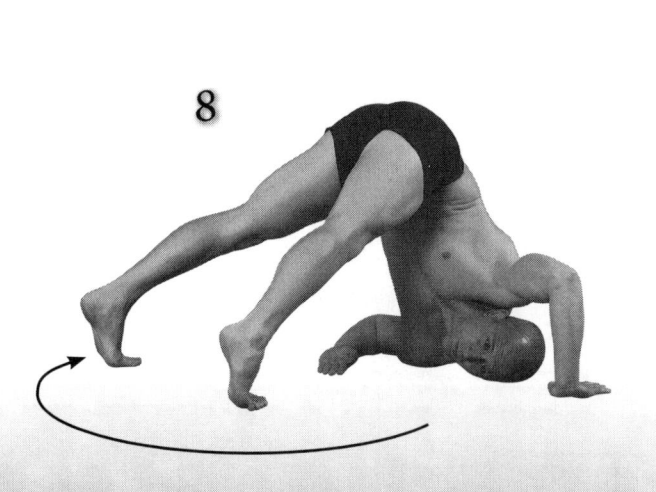

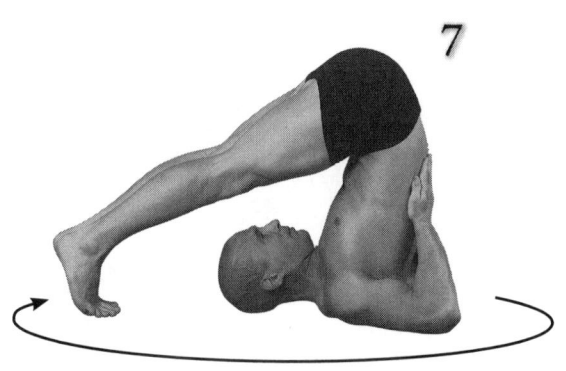

PRASARA YOGA: *Flow Beyond Thought*

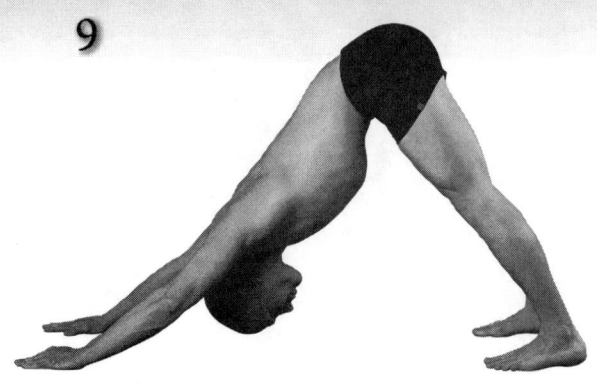

9

As you roll to face the ground, rise up into Downward-Facing Dog. Again, exhale and deepen into the pose as you are able (9).

You will now repeat the beginning sequence of Screwing Arms to Dolphin Pose (10–12), but now you will engage the Lateral Roll onto your left shoulder (13) to enter into the Plow (14).

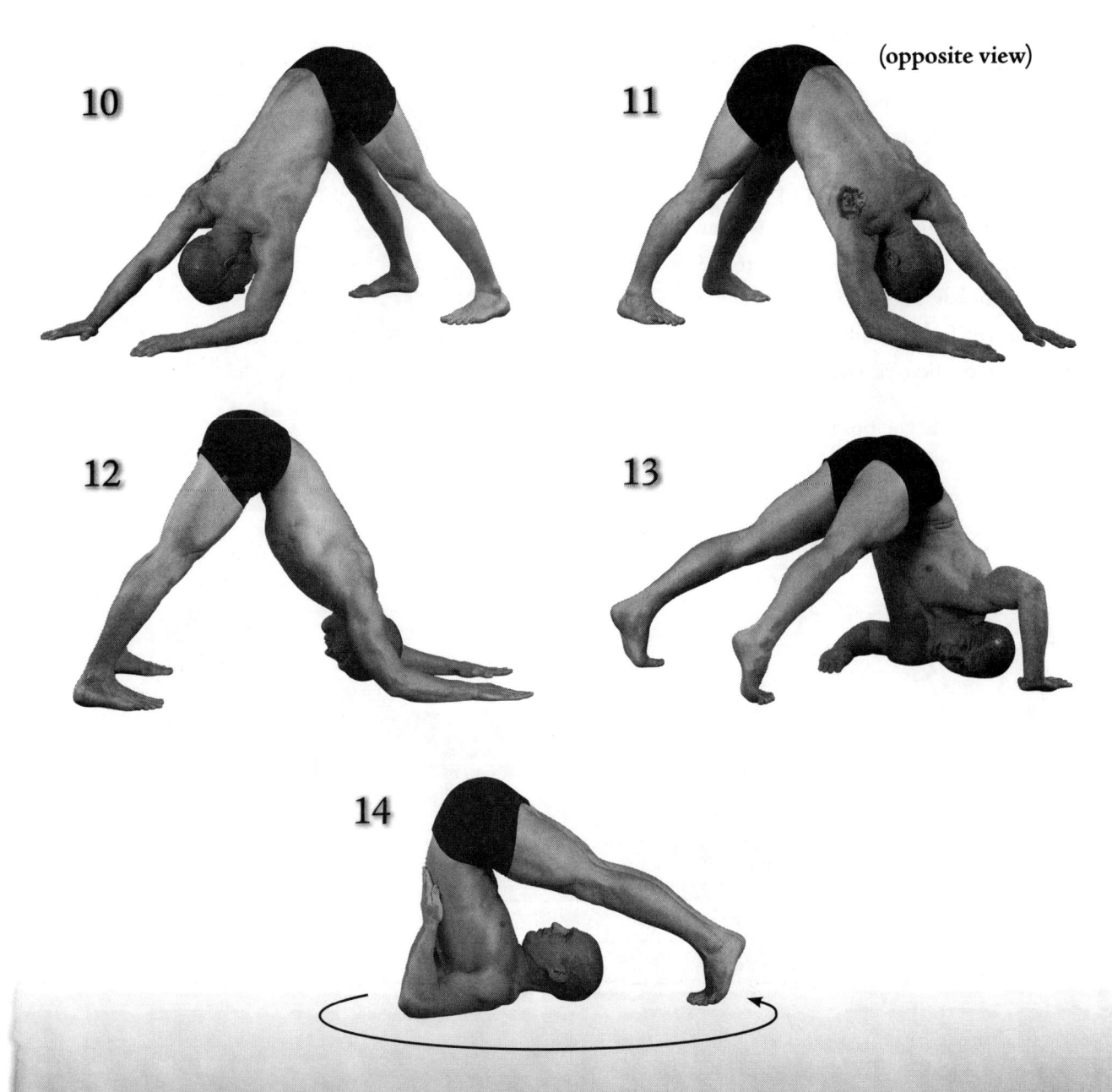

10

11 (opposite view)

12

13

14

132

PRASARA YOGA: *Flow Beyond Thought*

From the Plow, you will roll out onto your right shoulder (15) and into the Quad Squat (Manduka Asana). While on all fours, flatten your back and equally distribute the weight of your torso between all four limbs. Turn your hands inward while flaring your elbows and knees slightly outwards (16).

Inhale and exhale as you push up and raise your left leg up in the air to begin an Elevated Scorpion (17). In the Elevated Scorpion you lead with your knee as you bring it to the sky as high as you are able and reach the knee behind you and to your right side. Keep both hands firmly against the ground as you continue in this twist.

Eventually, you will reach the end range of your twist and the motion will bring your left hand off of the ground and you will support yourself strongly on your right hand and right foot. Your right leg will remain fully straight as you continue the movement. Reach fully and you will come to the end of the movement and land on the ball of your left foot.

Reach your left hand to the floor on the inside of your left knee and bring your right over to follow. You are now in the Side Lunge Pose (Parsva Anjaneyasana). Allow your hips to drop low and sink into this pose (18).

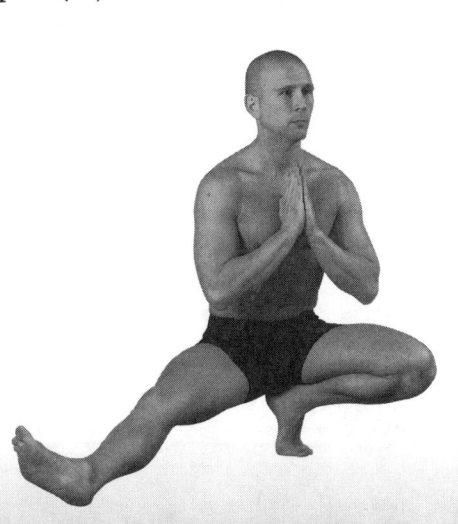

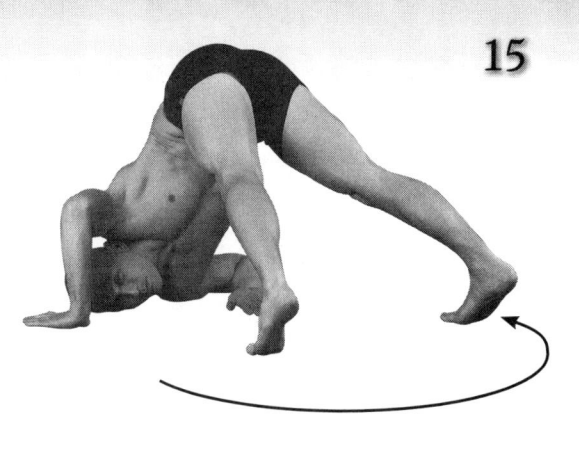

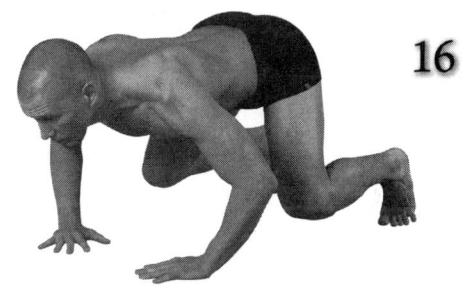

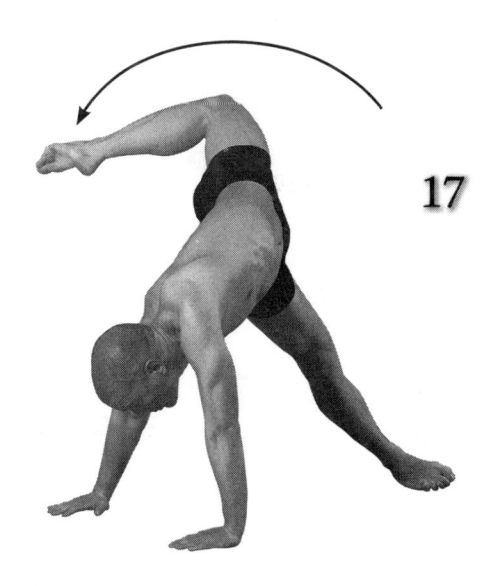

133

PRASARA YOGA: Flow Beyond Thought

19

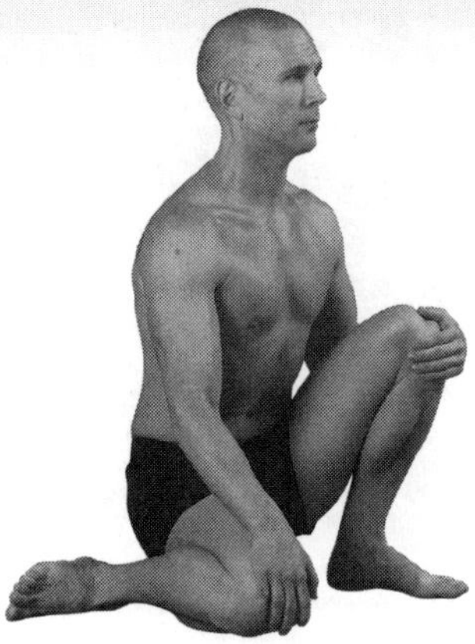

You will now roll your right foot down to the ground as you shift your weight and transition into the opposite Side Lunge Pose (19–21).

You are now in Side Lunge with your right knee bent and your left leg straight (22).

Swing your left leg out to the side to come back into the Quad Squat Position (23).

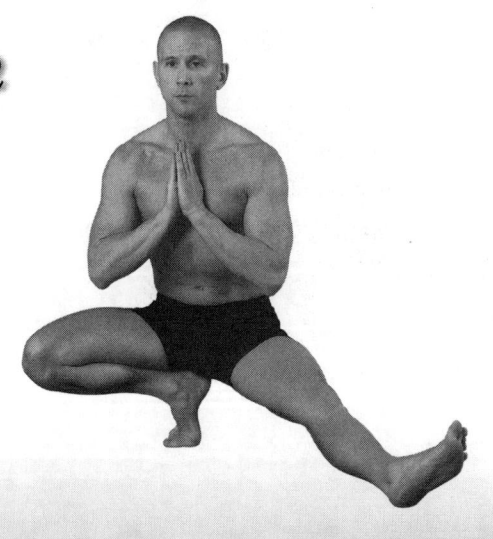

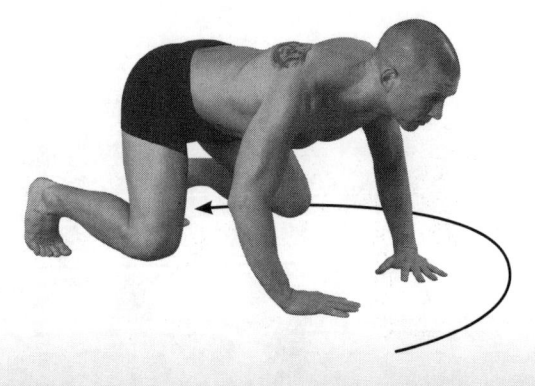

20

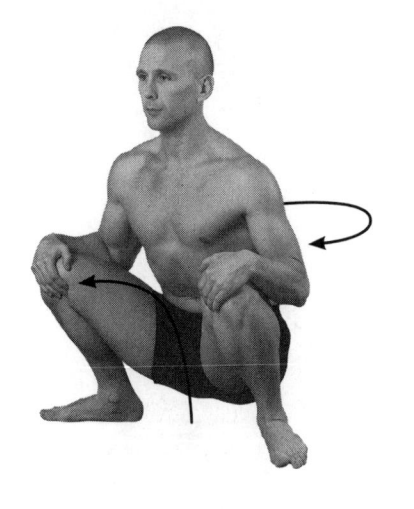

21

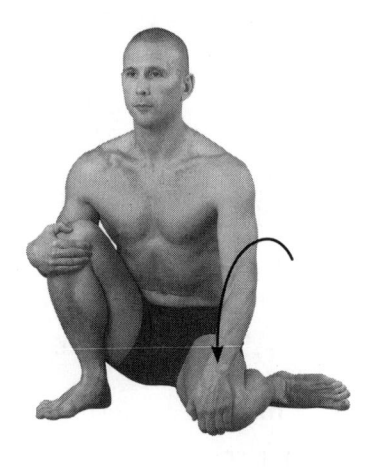

22

23

PRASARA YOGA: *Flow Beyond Thought*

Repeat the previous sequence into Elevated Scorpion, this time leading with the right leg up in the air (24).

This brings you to Side Lunge Pose with your left leg straight (25).

Inhale as you bring the left leg in toward your center to a Quad Squat Position (26) to prepare for the Crane Pose (Bakasana).

Exhale and widen your knees outwards slightly past your elbows. Keep the bend in your elbows and flare them outward to the side. You will now shift your weight slightly forward and, while on the balls of your feet, lay your knees on top of your bent arms just above the elbows. Bring your head forward and up to counter balance your weight, exhale to activate your core, and continue your forward lean. Find the balance point that will enable you to lift your feet off the floor. Keep your balance by pressing through your fingers and the heel of your palm. Your strong exhale will prime a good core activation and keep a solid hand balance (27).

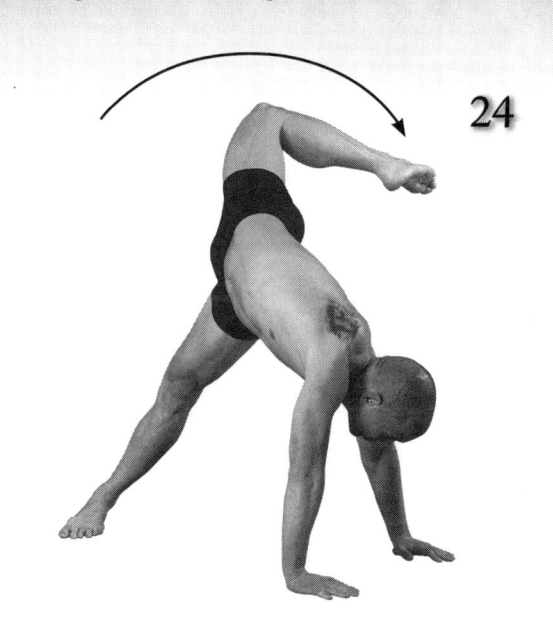

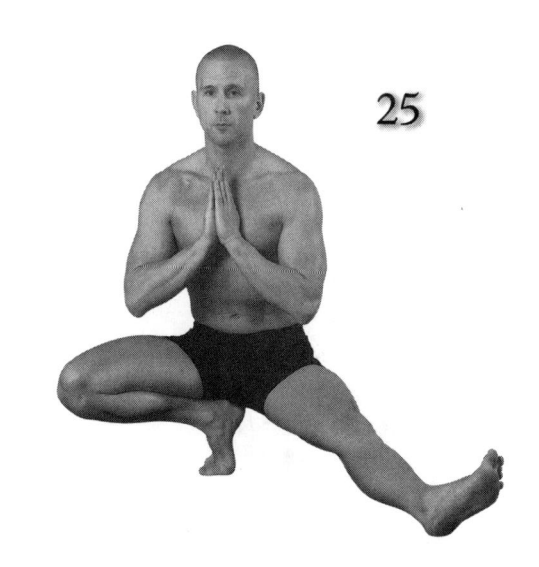

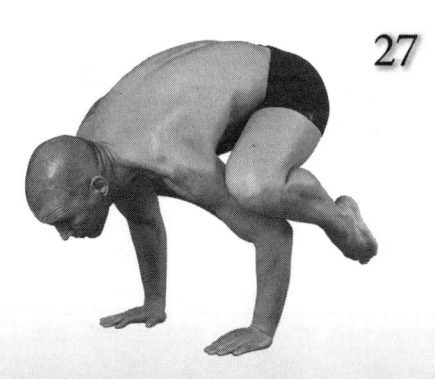

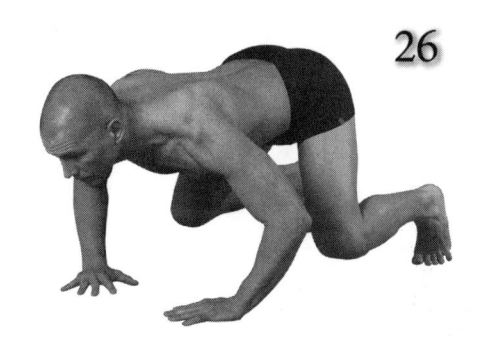

PRASARA YOGA: *Flow Beyond Thought*

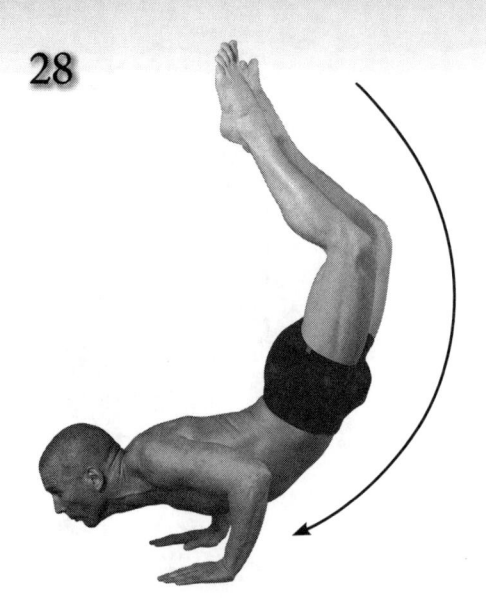

Inhale to prepare for a Spinal Wave to engage the ground. Exhale as you keep your arms fully stable and strongly bring your knees off your elbows to rise up in the air behind you (28).

Here is where you apply a strong hip snap and leg drive to roll the front of your body smoothly onto the ground.

As your chest and hips engage the ground, push firmly through your hands to straighten your elbows and finish in Upward-Facing Dog (Adho Mukha Svanasana). Turn your elbow pits forward and push against the floor, making sure not to shrug your shoulders up. Project your chest forward and up in front of you. Roll your shoulders back to engage in a strong shoulder pack. Look straight ahead or, if it is comfortable, lift your head and arch back to look at the sky. Squeeze your buttocks together and push your ankles into the floor. Exhale and sink into the pose to finish the Diving Dolphin flow (29).

TUMBLE WEED

PRASARA YOGA: Flow Beyond Thought

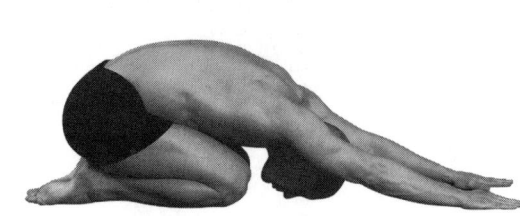

Tumbleweed begins in Sleeping Warrior Pose (Supta Vira Asana). Be firmly seated on your heels, keeping your knees together. Lean forward with good spinal alignment as you bring your torso forward and down to rest comfortably on your thighs. Exhale to fully seat yourself in the position and continue to keep your buttocks in contact with your heels. Reach forward with your palms flat on the ground to continue the feeling of your spine and upper body opening tall and long. Your forehead rests lightly on the ground (1).

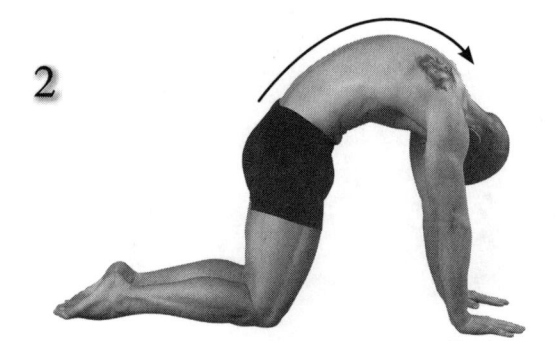

Inhale slightly as you push through your hands and lift your head up off the ground. Continue the lift by raising your hips and shifting them forward (2).

Exhale as your legs straighten and the front of your hips come down to the ground. You are now in Upward-Facing Dog (Urdhva Mukha Svanasana). Turn your elbow pits forward and push against the floor, bringing your shoulders down and away from your ears. Project your chest forward and up in front of you. Roll your shoulders back to engage in a strong shoulder pack. Look straight ahead. Squeeze your buttocks and thighs firmly and push your ankles into the floor (3).

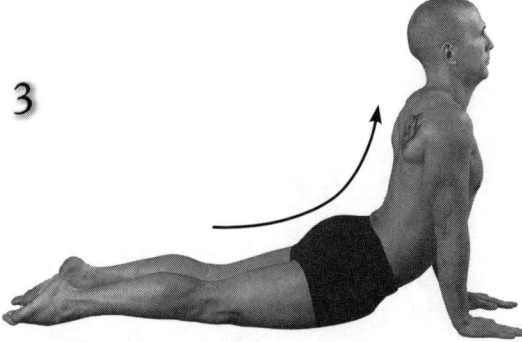

As you relax down toward Sphinx Pose (4), slow yourself down through the yielding strength of your core, contracting from the lower back. Minimize how much you press into the earth with your hands and forearms. To come out of Sphinx drop down and rest your chest and chin comfortably on the ground.

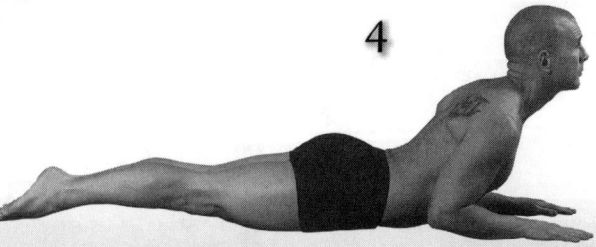

PRASARA YOGA: *Flow Beyond Thought*

Inhale through the nose as you arch your tailbone toward the sky into Caterpillar Pose A (5), and drive your elbows back until your forearms touch the earth. Arch the fan of connective tissue across your lower back in a tight circle around toward the back of your head.

Exhale as you release the whip of A into Caterpillar Pose B (6) by tucking your tailbone back underneath. Continue the string of pearls motion on your spine as you round your mid-back toward the sky, and exhale as you move your navel toward your spine and contract the corset of muscle around your core. Keep your strong arms driving the earth away, but pull your elbows tightly to the sides of your rib cage. Be strong and squeeze everything out to restore the floating nest of connective tissue that holds your organs healthily in gravity.

Inhale to release and roll first the top of your thighs and then your hips back down into the earth as you move back into Sphinx Pose (7). Roll the shoulders back, arching from the lower back to lift your crown upwards. Drive your elbows back but minimize how much you press into the ground to elevate.

Exhale as you extend your elbows to locked position and drive the earth away. Contract your glutes to release your hips into the ground. Zip up your knees and find the top of your feet to drive your hips toward your wrists. Lift your chest toward the sky for full Upward-Facing Dog Pose (8.)

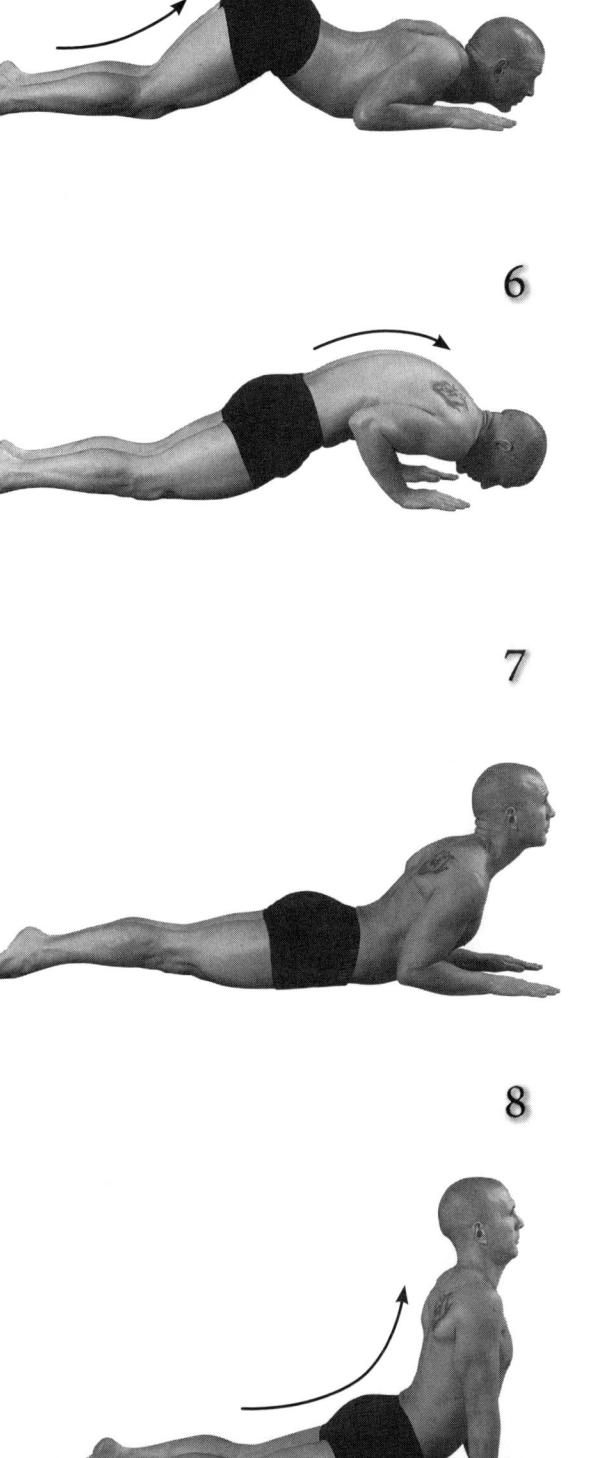

PRASARA YOGA: Flow Beyond Thought

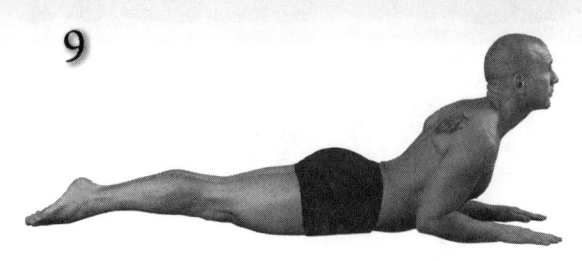

Relax your position by bending your elbows to come down to the floor (9); roll onto your right shoulder and bring your left knee up towards your body to flex your hips to slightly past 90 degrees.

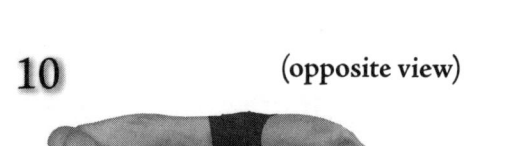

Plant your left foot firmly on the ground as you raise your hips and thread your right leg through and under your supporting left leg (10). The ability to push with your legs is very important in this pose.

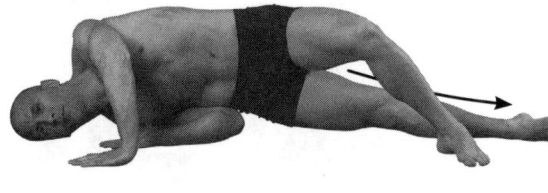

Start the upward push of this pose by pushing off through the midfoot, contracting your buttocks and hips to rise up toward the sky. Now, bring your hands behind your hips to lift up further. Your weight will be distributed between your upper back and shoulders. You are now in Shoulder Bridge (Setu Bandha Sarvangasana). Exhale with a relaxed throat and strive for that nice curve from the back of your neck to your hips (11).

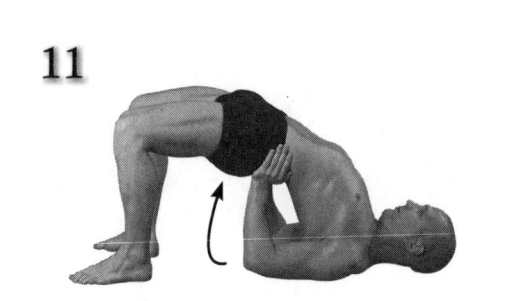

Flow smoothly out of the pose by dropping your hips and rolling onto your left shoulder. Keep firmly on your right foot as you bend the left leg and thread it through and under your right leg (12). Continue to bring your leg straight and in line with your hips and upper body.

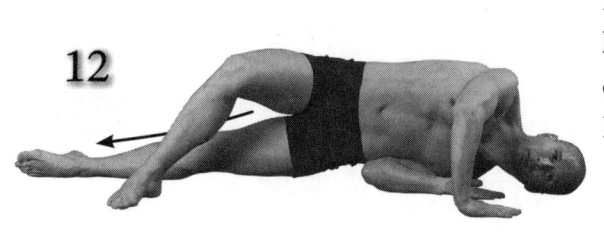

Next, bring your right leg next to your left leg and lie fully prone with your hands underneath the front of your shoulders (13). Press firmly up into Upward-Facing Dog (14).

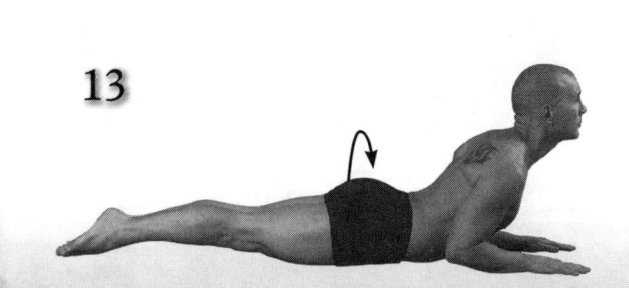

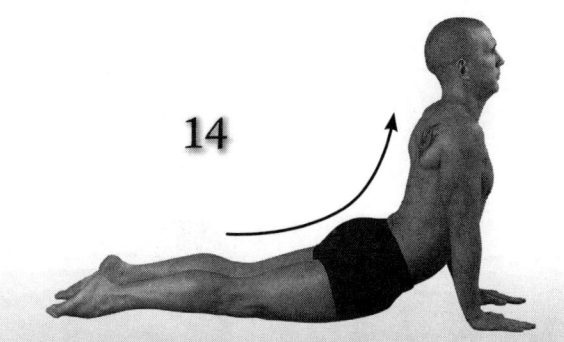

140

PRASARA YOGA: *Flow Beyond Thought*

You will now repeat the sequence of dropping onto the right shoulder to thread your legs to Shoulder Bridge Pose (15–17).

Then transition smoothly again to Upward-Facing Dog (18–21). Push firmly through your hands as you tuck your chin and shift your hips back and settle into Sleeping Warrior Pose (22). This concludes the first kinetic chain.

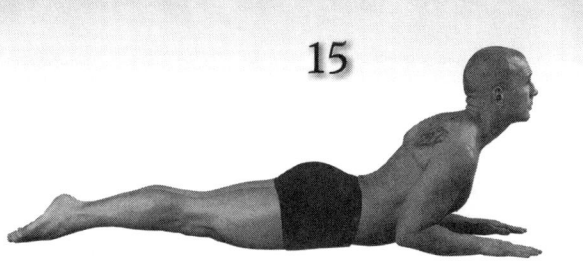

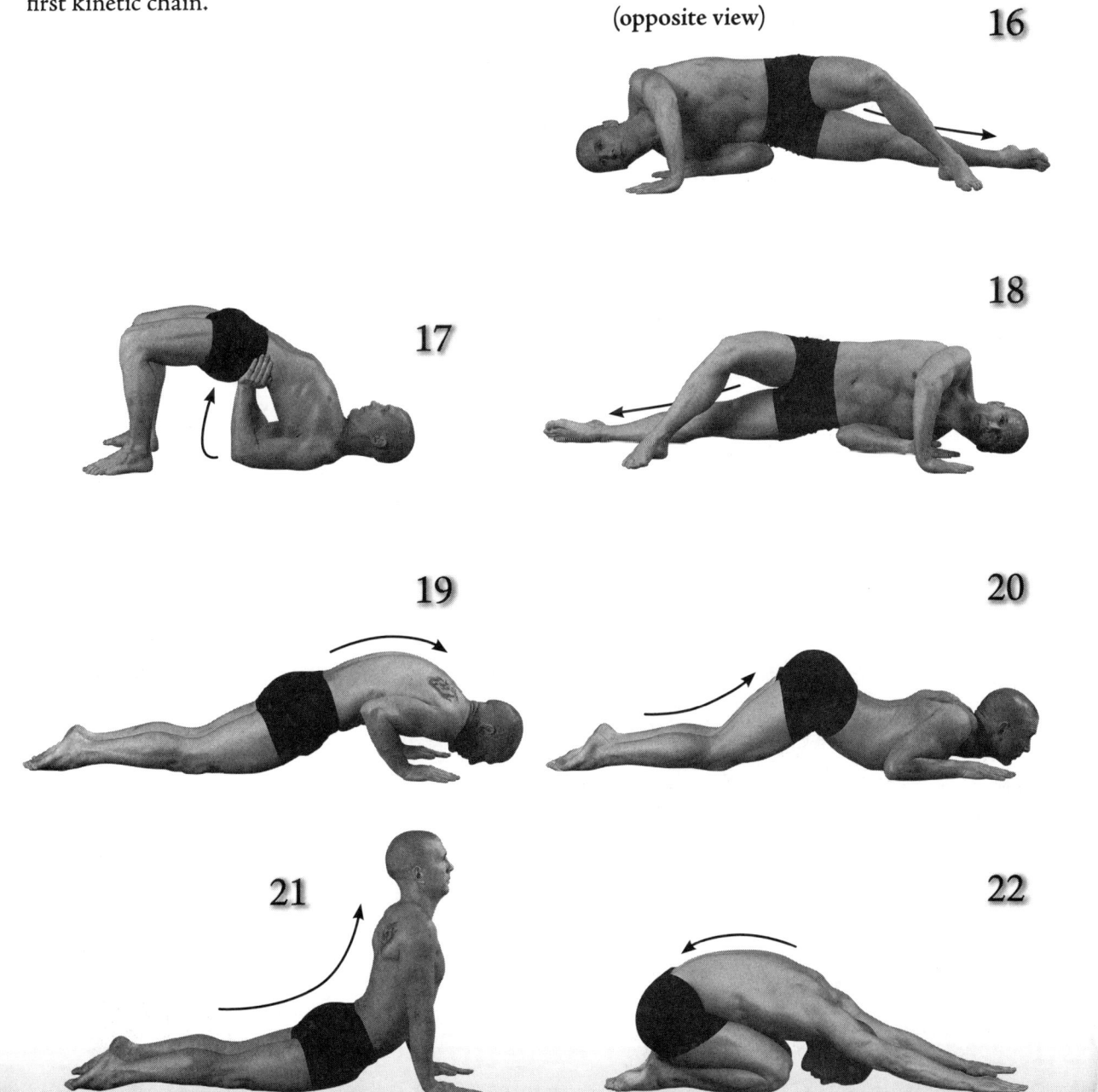

(opposite view)

PRASARA YOGA: *Flow Beyond Thought*

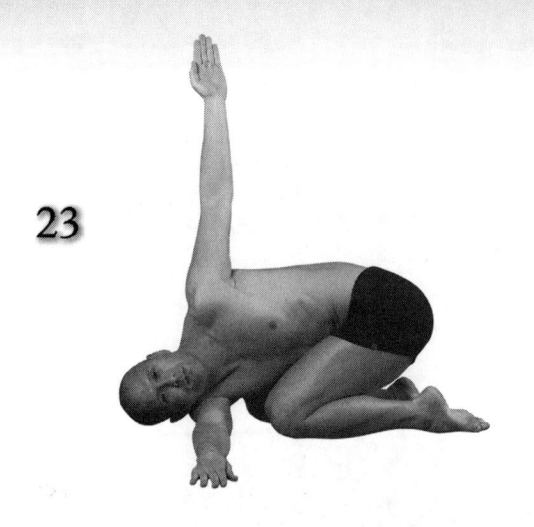

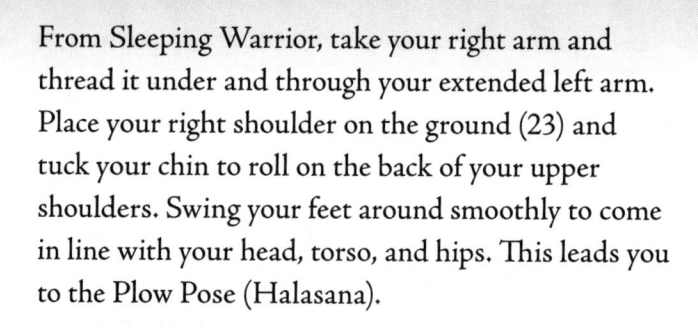

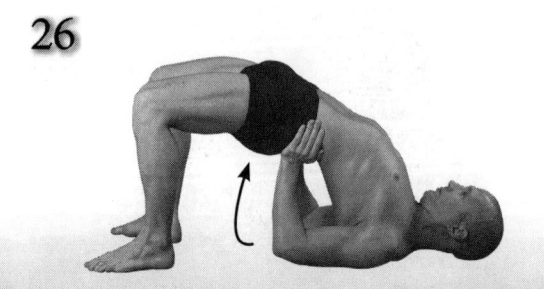

From Sleeping Warrior, take your right arm and thread it under and through your extended left arm. Place your right shoulder on the ground (23) and tuck your chin to roll on the back of your upper shoulders. Swing your feet around smoothly to come in line with your head, torso, and hips. This leads you to the Plow Pose (Halasana).

Focus on keeping your legs straight and lifting the back of your knees and your hips toward the sky. It helps to think of pushing your chest out and away. This will keep you in proper alignment. Exhale fully as you relax your neck and throat to deepen into the pose (24).

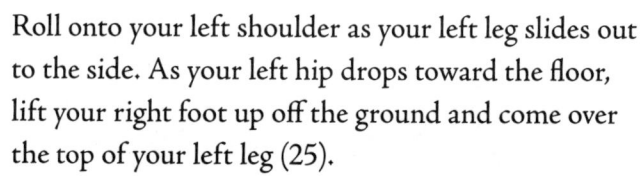

Roll onto your left shoulder as your left leg slides out to the side. As your left hip drops toward the floor, lift your right foot up off the ground and come over the top of your left leg (25).

Continue the movement to pivot around your hips and arrive firmly in Shoulder Bridge (26).

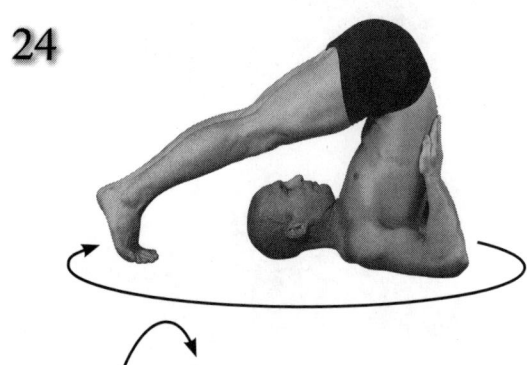

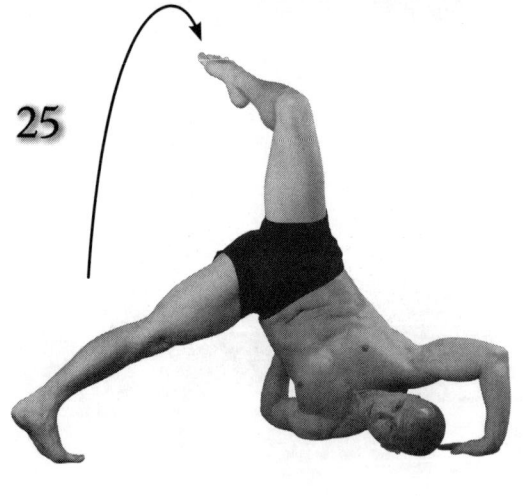

PRASARA YOGA: *Flow Beyond Thought*

You will now transition out of this posture by lifting your left arm up and placing your palm down on the floor above your head (27). Take your right arm in the opposite direction toward your feet.

Continue the motion and roll onto your right shoulder, pushing firmly through your left foot as you pivot around the back of your upper shoulders. Again, not on the back of your head! This is called a Twisting Spinal Arch.

Bring your right leg up over the top of your left leg as you pivot and you will arrive in the Plow (28). Remember always to exhale fully to surrender into the posture.

Flow smoothly out of the Plow by swinging your left leg out away from your right leg. This will have you rolling on your left shoulder with your left arm across your chest between you and the ground. Bring your knees together and sink your stomach down onto your thighs (29). You are now in a position to move seamlessly back into Plow, rolling on the left shoulder and onto your upper back. As you bring your legs around into position, keep your throat relaxed and allow your body to compress the air from your lungs, and be breathed by the motion (30).

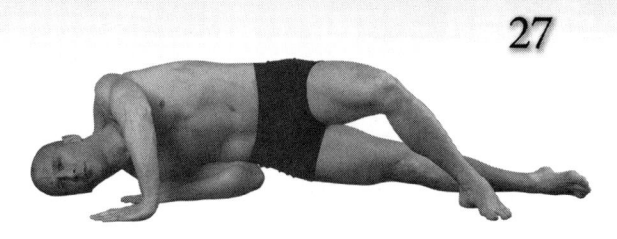

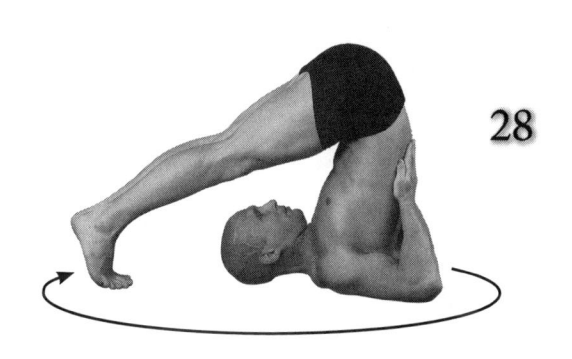

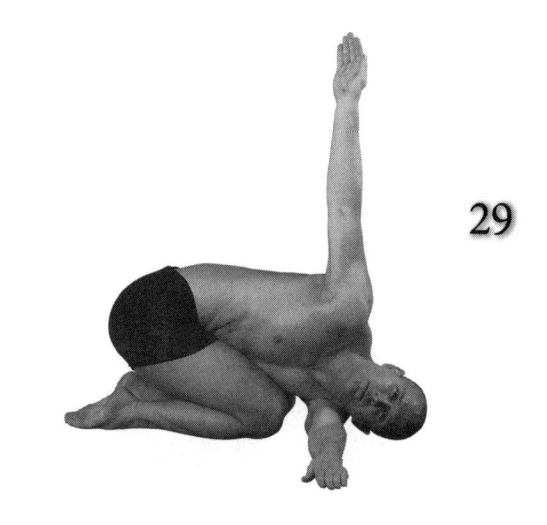

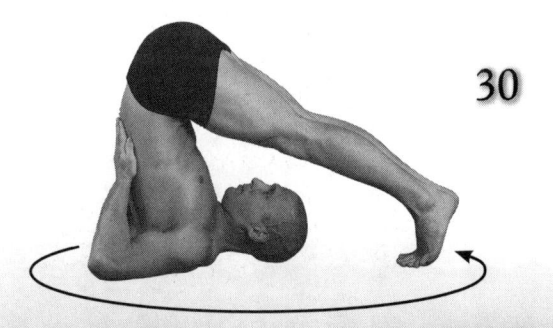

143

PRASARA YOGA: *Flow Beyond Thought*

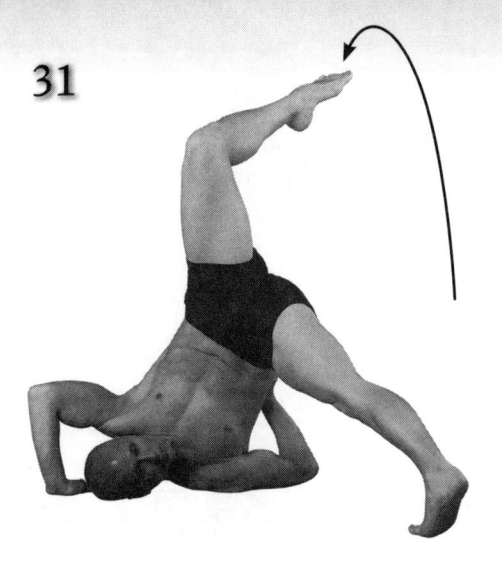

31

Repeat the transition sequence into Shoulder Bridge by continuing the motion onto your right shoulder, pressing firmly through your right leg as the left leg comes up and over into the position (31).

Lift your hips up strongly to engage in a nice Shoulder Bridge (32).

Bringing your right hand up and your left hand down starts the last Twisting Spinal Arch out of Shoulder Bridge toward the final Plow.

Now, bring your right leg over your left as you pivot on your upper back. Exhale smoothly into a firm Plow Position. Continue the roll onto your left shoulder and bring your knees together to Child's Pose. This ends the second kinetic chain (33–35).

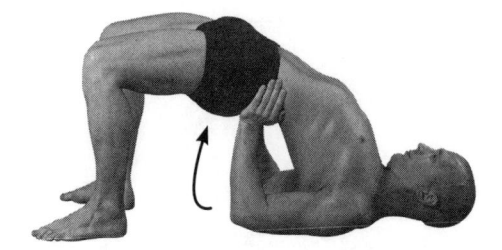

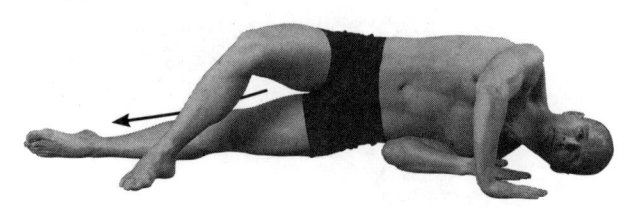

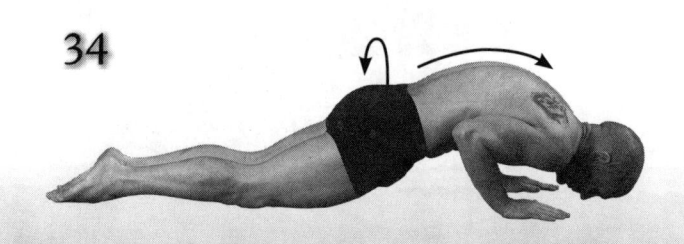

32

33

34

PRASARA YOGA: *Flow Beyond Thought*

From Child's Pose, extend your left leg straight behind you and roll smoothly to the right onto your back (36).

As your back contacts the ground, bring your left heel close into your buttock and reach your left hand down to grasp your left ankle (37).

This is a Long Leg Roll. Bring your right heel toward your buttock as well as you place your right hand across and above your head to your left-hand side. Exhale fully to lift your hips up high to be supported through your feet and your left shoulder. This is a Single Shoulder Bridge. Open your chest up and out, contracting your glutes strongly to fully open the right side of your body (37).

Drop your hips down as you roll to your right and bring your right knee in toward your chest. Bring your knees together to flow briefly through Child's Pose. Rather than stopping in this pose, straighten your right leg back behind you immediately and continue a Long Leg Roll onto your left side (38).

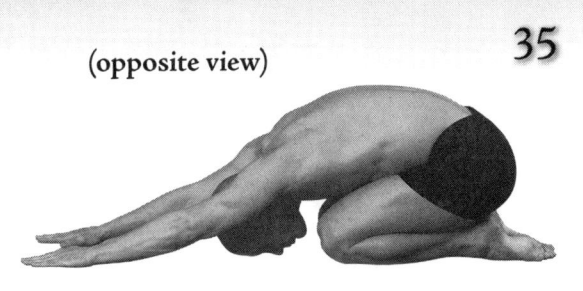

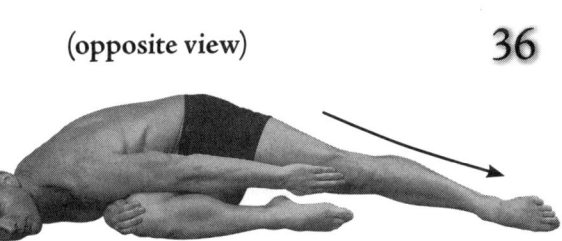

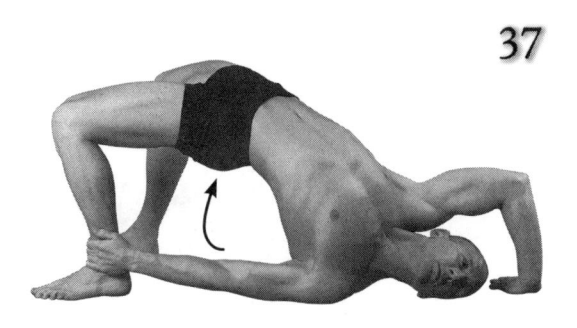

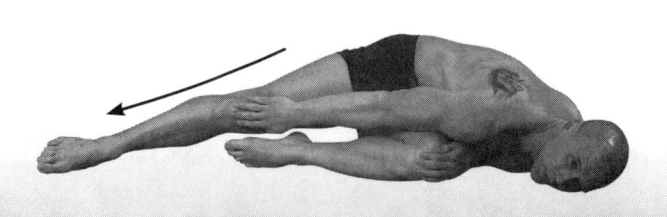

(opposite view) 35

(opposite view) 36

37

38

PRASARA YOGA: *Flow Beyond Thought*

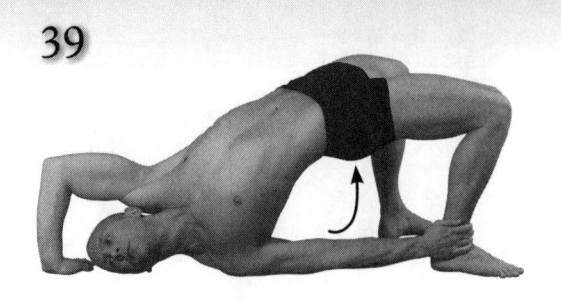

39

You will now engage in the Single Shoulder Bridge onto your right side. Remember to bring your heels close to your buttocks as you grasp your right ankle with your right hand (39). Take your left hand across and over your head to your right-hand side. Lift your hips strongly and exhale to fully open the left side of your body.

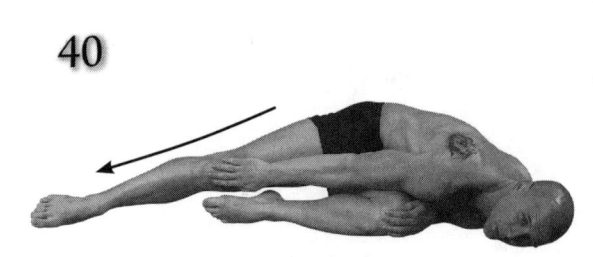

Bring your hips down out of the pose as you bring your left knee in toward your chest (40). This allows you to roll smoothly to your left, bringing your knees together to finish in Child's Pose and concluding the Tumbleweed flow (41).

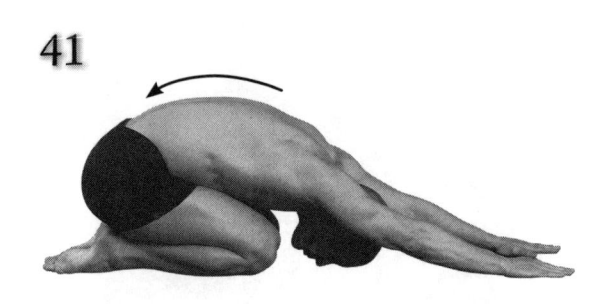

40

41

146

FLOCK OF PIGEONS

PRASARA YOGA: *Flow Beyond Thought*

1

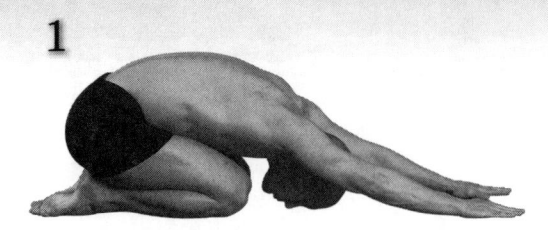

Flock of Pigeons flow begins in Child's Pose (Balasana). Be firmly seated on your heels and slightly separate your knees. With a straight back, deliberately bring your chest and stomach forward and down to rest comfortably on your thighs (1).

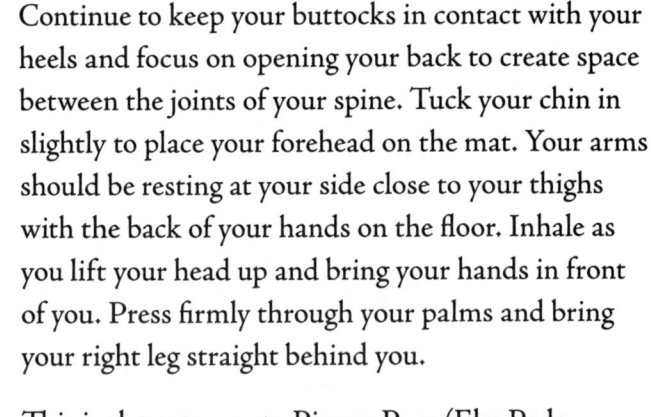

Continue to keep your buttocks in contact with your heels and focus on opening your back to create space between the joints of your spine. Tuck your chin in slightly to place your forehead on the mat. Your arms should be resting at your side close to your thighs with the back of your hands on the floor. Inhale as you lift your head up and bring your hands in front of you. Press firmly through your palms and bring your right leg straight behind you.

2

This is the entrance to Pigeon Pose (Eka Pada Rajakapotasana). Straighten your right leg behind you while keeping your left shin perpendicular to your torso (2). Think of making your right leg as long as possible with the top of your foot flat against the ground. Roll the front of your right hip inwards into the floor while keeping your shoulders squarely pointed toward the front. Squeeze your right buttock. Your torso should be upright and tall, maintaining the proper crown-to-coccyx alignment. Exhale and sink deeply into the posture.

The transition to the opposite Pigeon Pose begins with placing your hands down for support as you swing your right leg in front and place it next to your left knee to come to a Triangle Squat (3).

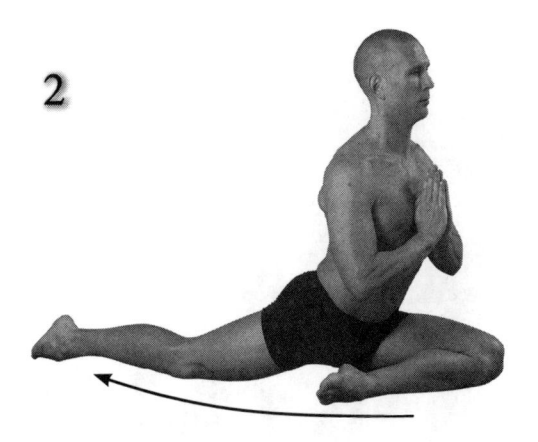

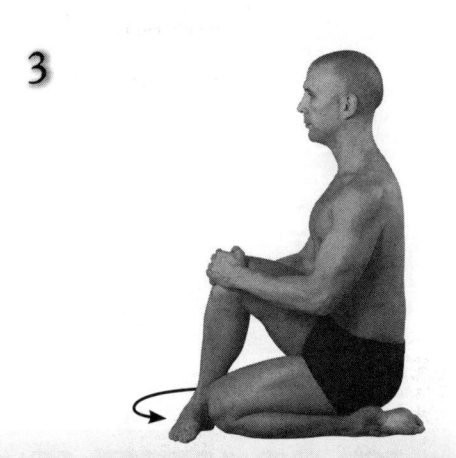

3

(opposite view)

148

PRASARA YOGA: *Flow Beyond Thought*

Continue turning to the left as you complete a Standing Shin Roll by lifting your left knee up to the side (4) and turning on your heel as your right knee comes down to the ground. You will find yourself in the opposite side Triangle Squat (5).

Continue to turn by pivoting through the middle of your right shin as your left leg swings back behind you to finish in Pigeon Pose with your left leg straight (6). Again, breathe out fully to go deeply into the pose.

You will then simply repeat the process to return to Pigeon Pose with your right leg back behind you (7–10). Next, bring your right leg up and bring your knees in together to Child's Pose (11). This completes the first kinetic chain of Flock of Pigeons.

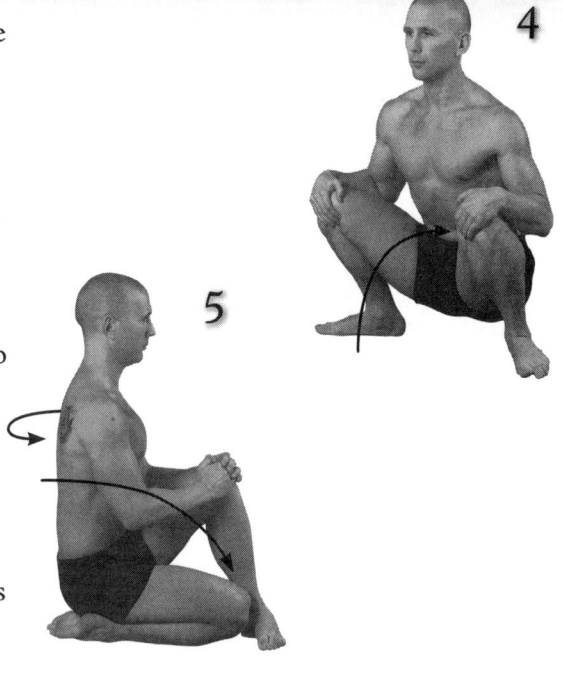

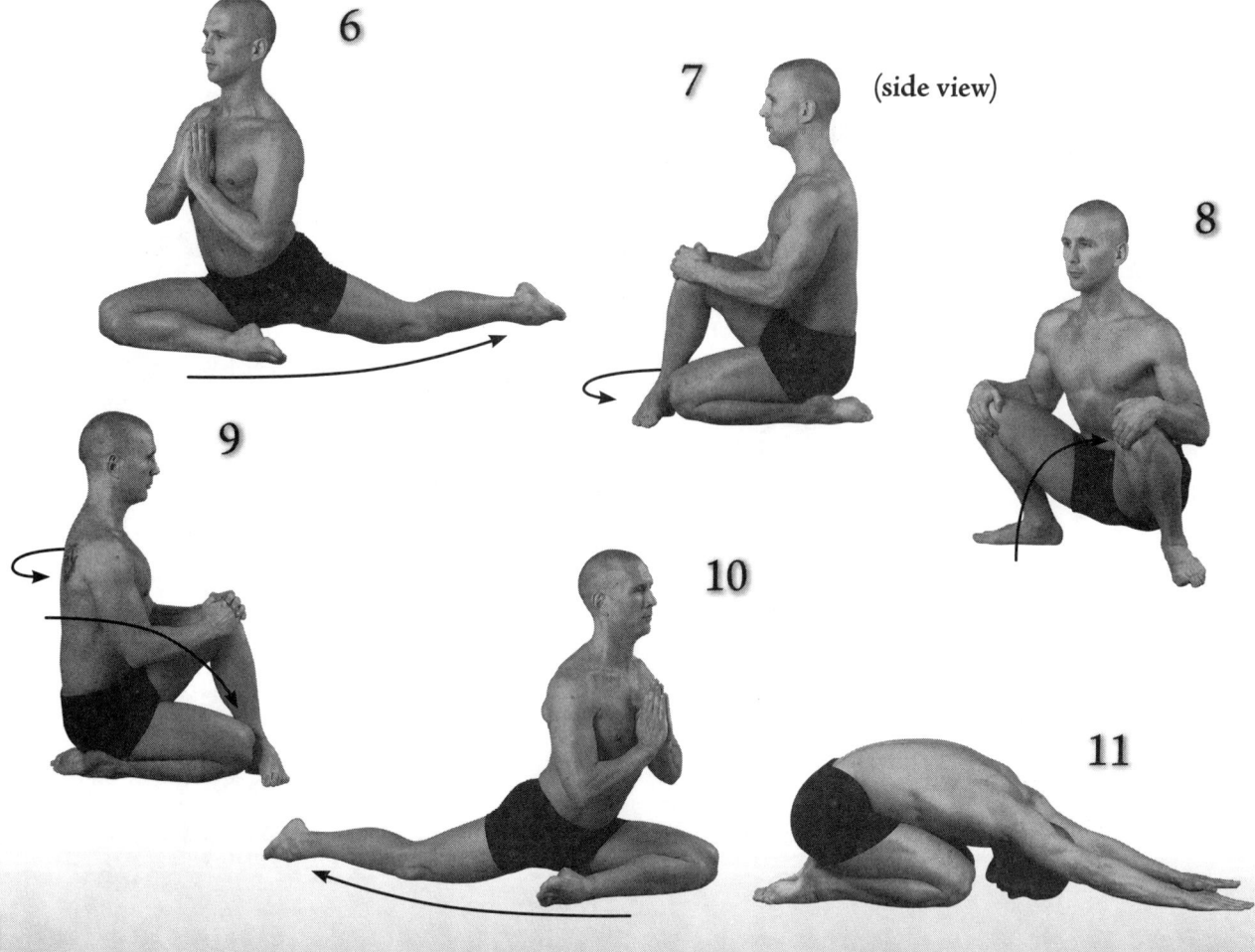

(side view)

149

PRASARA YOGA: *Flow Beyond Thought*

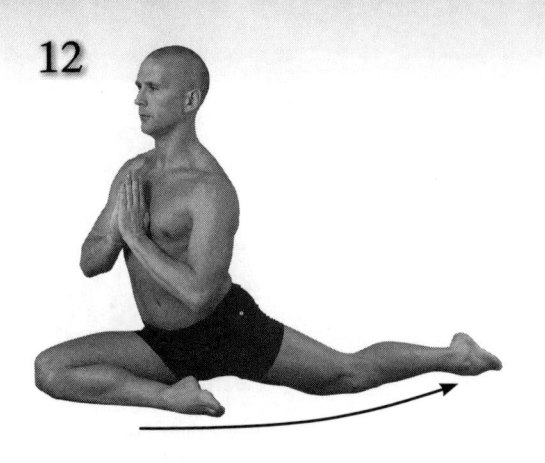

The second kinetic chain of the flow begins in Pigeon Pose with the left leg back. The transition to the opposite Pigeon Pose is now achieved by swinging your left leg around from the side (13) to start a Double Shin Roll.

Bring your left leg straight in front of you and place your heel down with your toes pointed (14). Shift your hips as you roll forward onto your left shin and your right leg straightens back behind you to finish in Pigeon Pose (15).

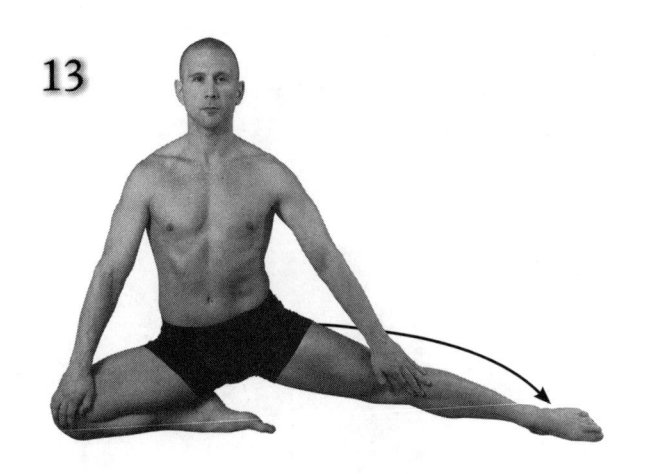

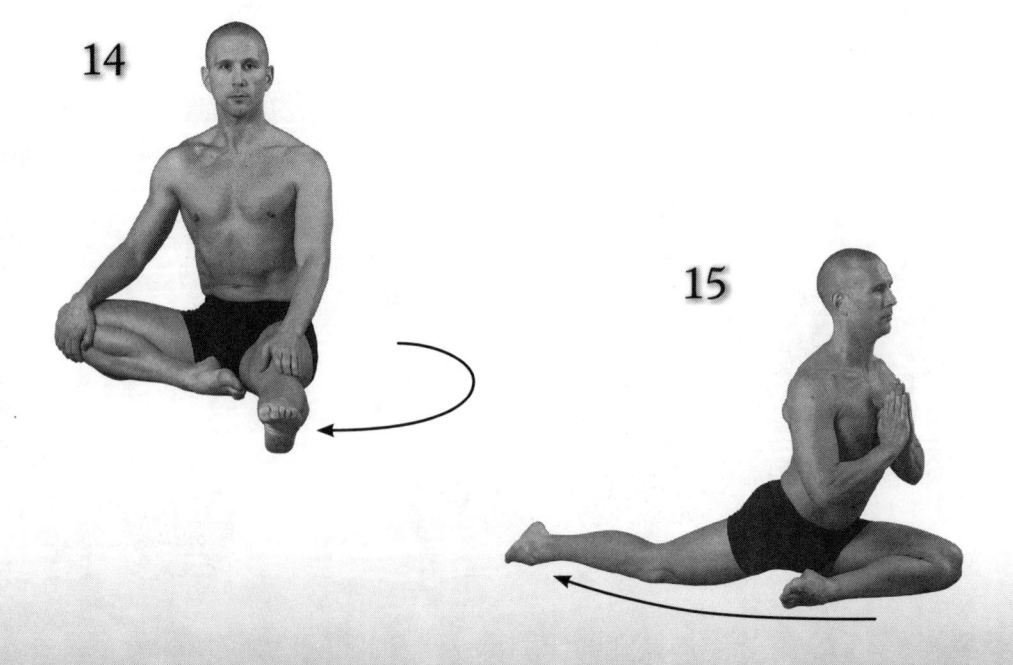

PRASARA YOGA: *Flow Beyond Thought*

Inhale as you lean forward and place your hands on the ground. Exhale and push firmly to bring your left knee up into Lunge Pose (Anjaneyasana). Your hips and shoulders should be square to face forward as your hands rest on top of your left knee. Be tall, projecting your chest forward and up. You should be engaging in a good hip snap and leg drive to push your hips forward and open the front of your right thigh, your right buttock contracting firmly. Exhale fully for good core activation to be strong and stable in your upper body, allowing your lower body to surrender (16).

The transition to the opposite Lunge Pose begins by shifting your upper body forward onto your left thigh and bending your right knee to bring your right heel closer to you. The inside of your right shin will contact the ground (17) and you can shift your weight smoothly onto your right heel as you bring your right knee up in the air (18). This is called a Knee Switch. As your right knee comes up, your left knee goes down to the ground (19). Continue to turn until your left kneecap is placed on the ground and you finish in the Lunge Pose with your left leg back (20). Again, exhale fully with good alignment to now fully open the front of your left leg.

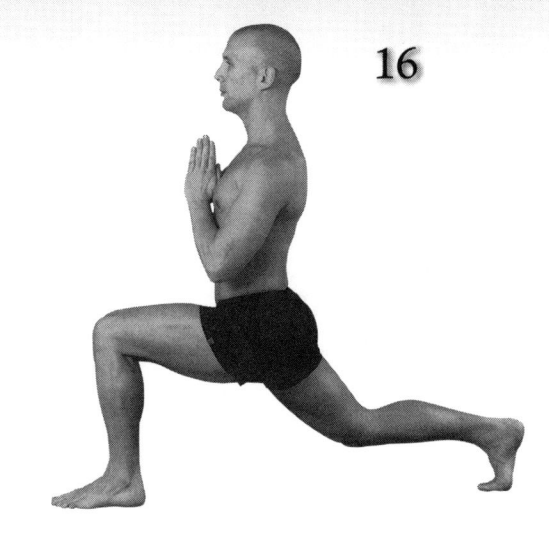

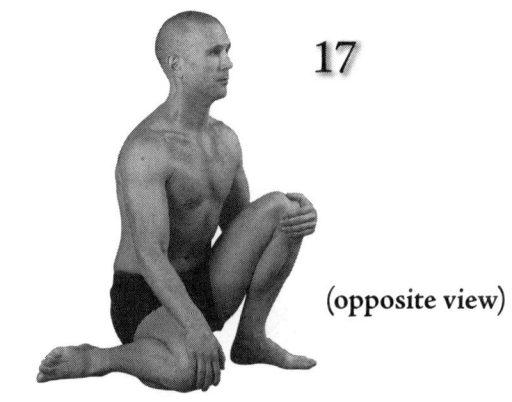

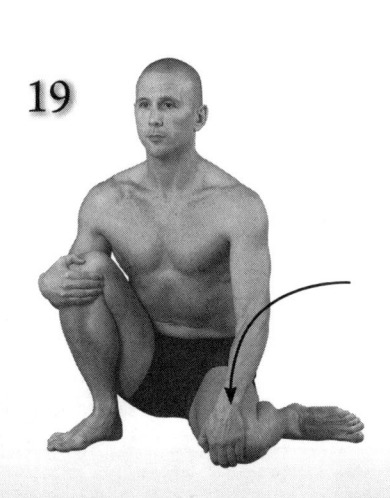

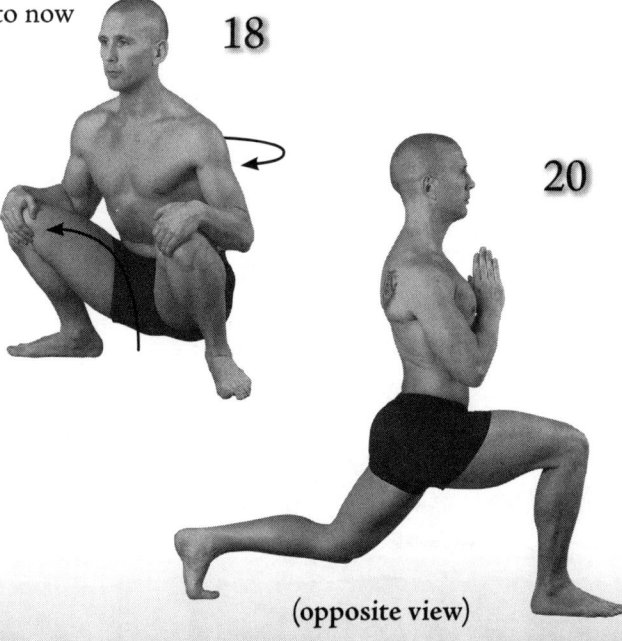

(opposite view)

(opposite view)

PRASARA YOGA: *Flow Beyond Thought*

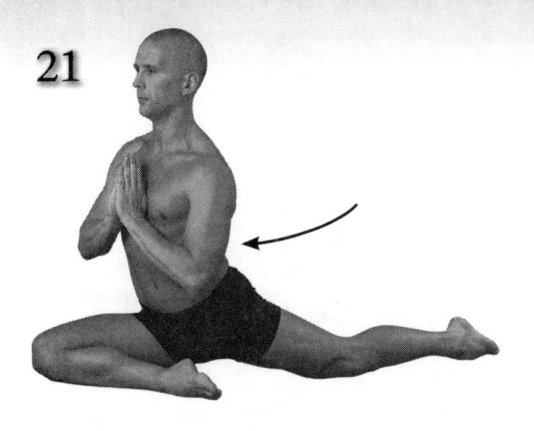

Lean your upper body forward and place your hands down on the ground; this will allow you to smoothly bring the side of your right knee down to engage in another Pigeon Pose (21).

Repeat the first movement of this second kinetic chain by bringing your left leg in front of you for another Double Shin Roll (22–23). Flow freely into Pigeon Pose with your right leg back (24). Then shift to the Lunge Pose with your right leg back (25).

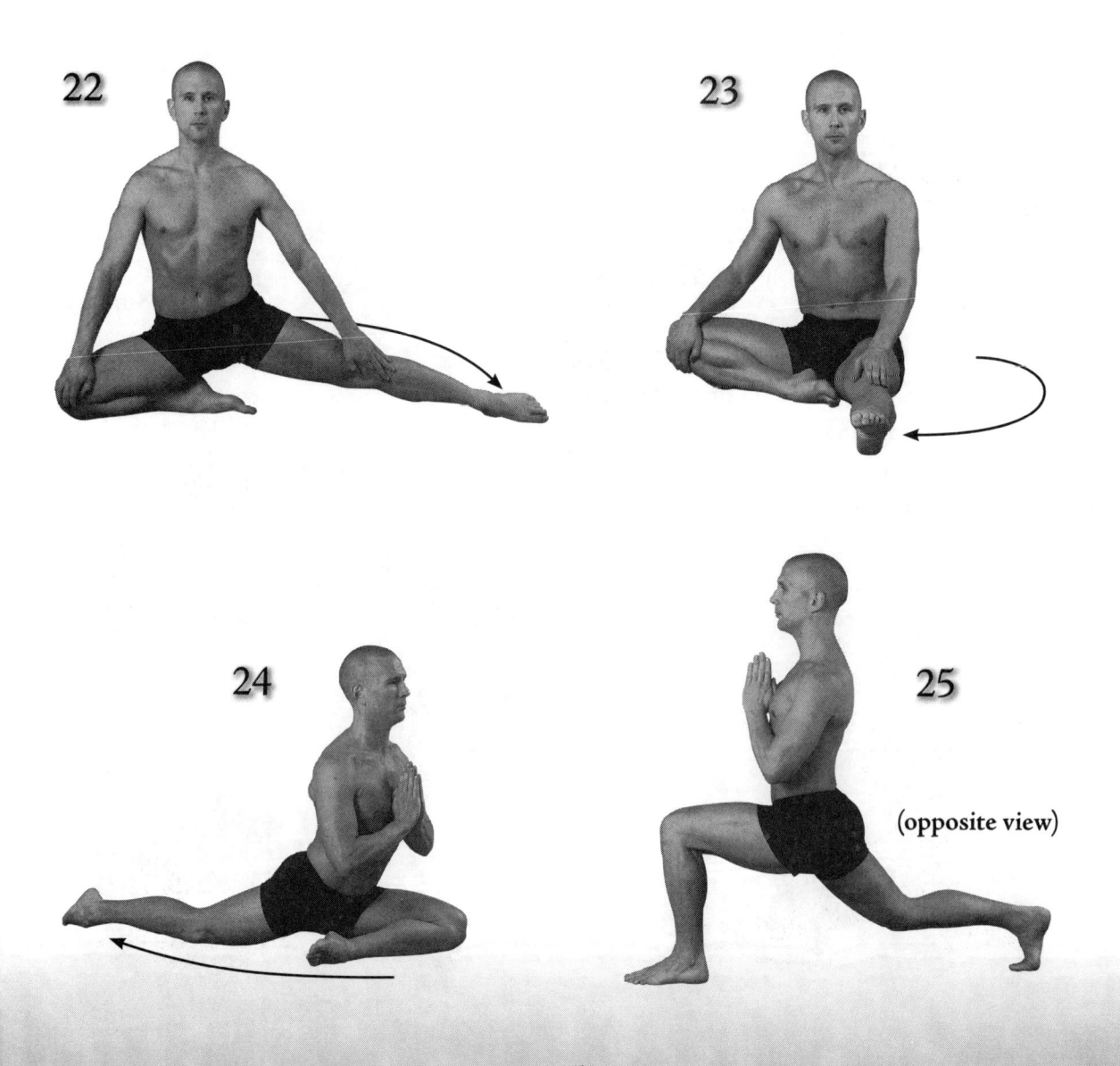

(opposite view)

PRASARA YOGA: *Flow Beyond Thought*

Continue on by flowing into another Knee Switch (26–28) to bring your right knee up into a nice, deep Lunge Pose with the left leg back (29). Drop your right knee down to a final Pigeon Pose (30) and bring your left knee up together with your right knee to finish in Child's Pose (31). This finishes the second kinetic chain of Flock of Pigeons.

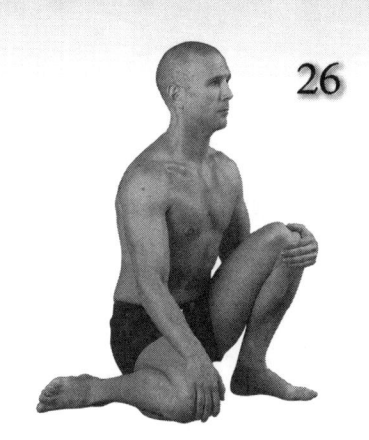

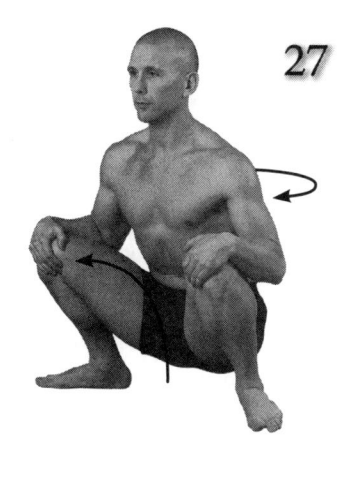

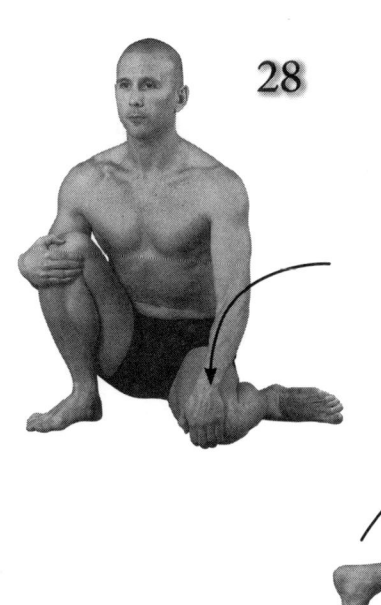

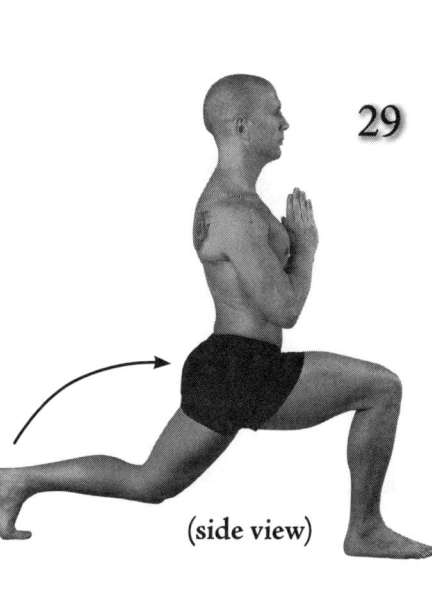

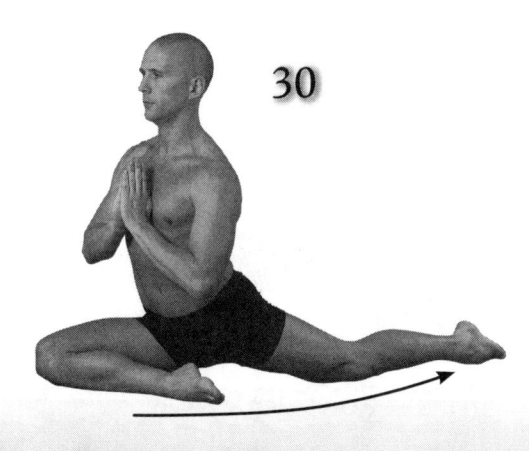

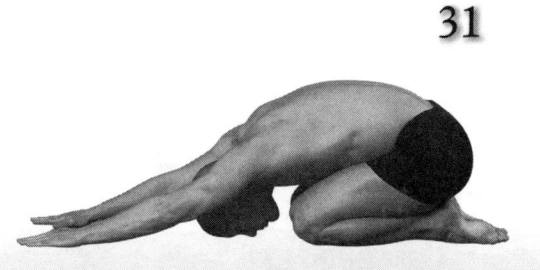

(side view)

PRASARA YOGA: *Flow Beyond Thought*

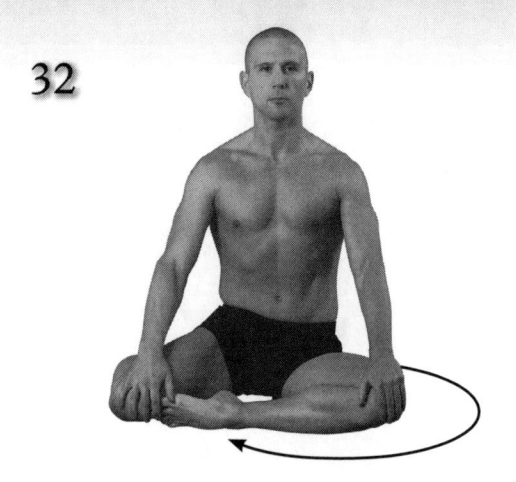

32

The last section of this flow starts with placing your right leg behind you out of Child's Pose. The inside of your right knee contacts the ground as your left shin is tucked close into your right thigh (32).

Sit on your buttocks as you shift to your right. The right knee will come up and out to your side as your left knee comes up off the floor. This is a Shinbox Switch (33).

Continue the motion until the outside of your right knee comes down to the ground and the inside of your left knee does the same (34).

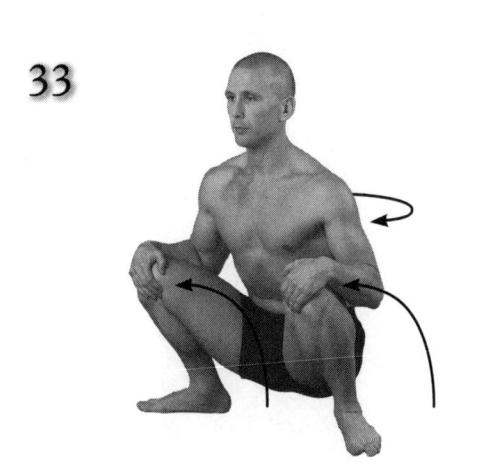

As you turn, snake your left hand to the inside of your left ankle and grasp the top of your foot. Bring your foot in toward your buttocks as you continue to shift forward onto your right shin. Maintain proper crown-to-coccyx alignment and you will arrive in King Pigeon Pose (35). Always remember to exhale into the pose; this will allow you to fully engage in the correct posture.

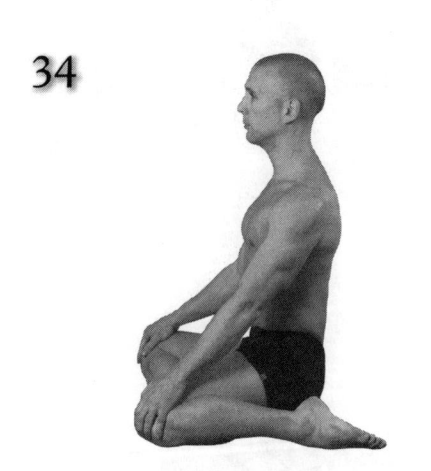

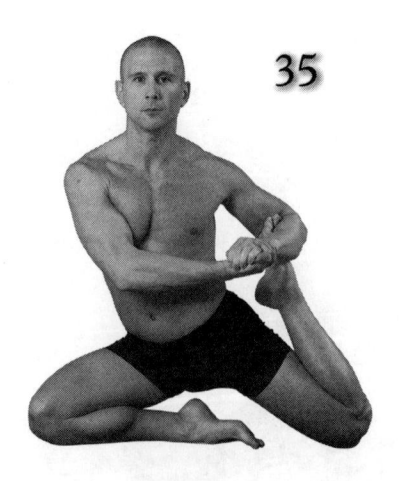

33

34

35

(front view)

PRASARA YOGA: *Flow Beyond Thought*

You will then reverse the Shinbox Switch (36–38) as you transition to the opposite King Pigeon Pose, with your right hand grasping your right foot (39).

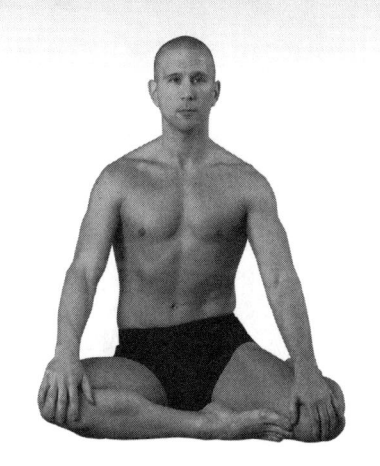

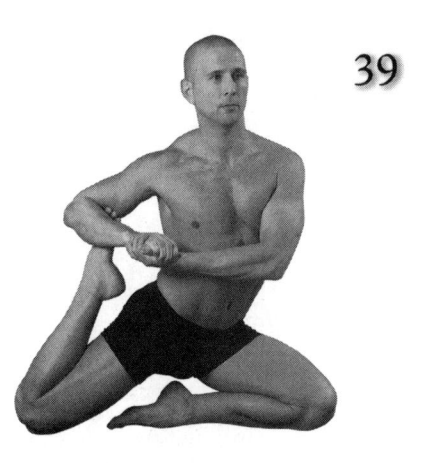

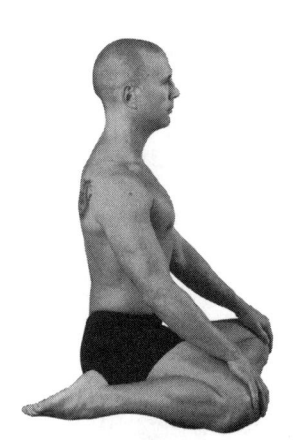

36

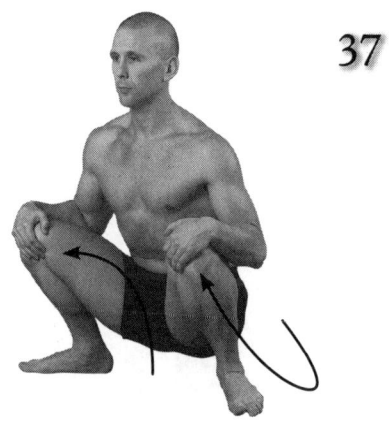

37

39

38

155

PRASARA YOGA: *Flow Beyond Thought*

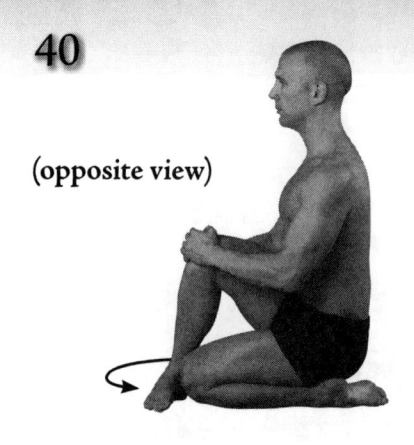

40

(opposite view)

The next step is a smooth flow that begins with the Triangle Squat transition that you performed in the first kinetic chain (40–43). However, instead of finishing in the opposite Pigeon Pose, you will continue to the Shinbox Switch transition and finish in King Pigeon Pose with your right leg back (44). You have essentially flowed out of the King Pigeon Pose and moved back into the same pose.

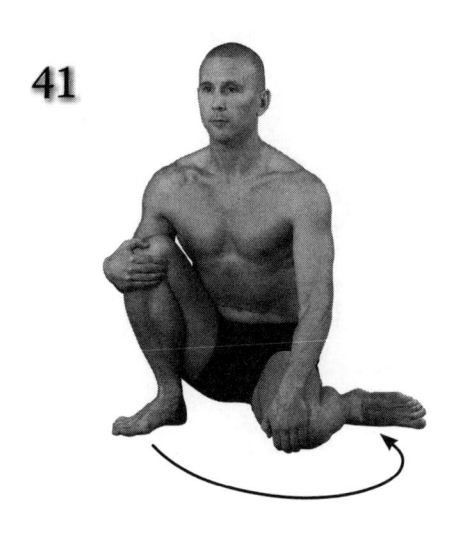

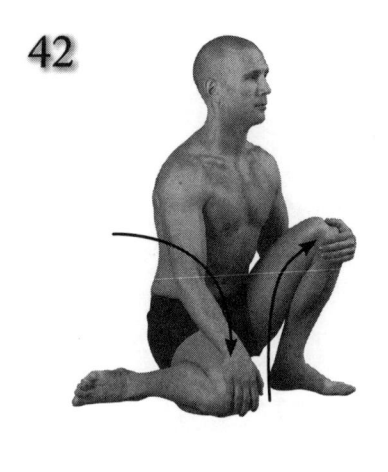

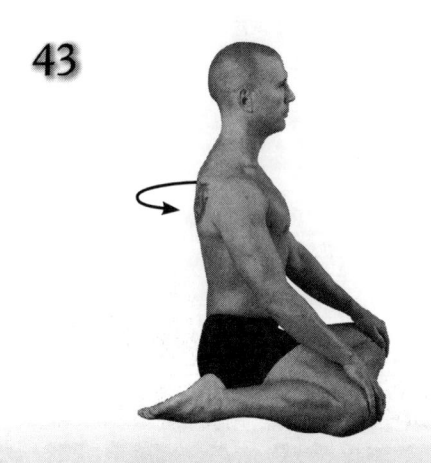

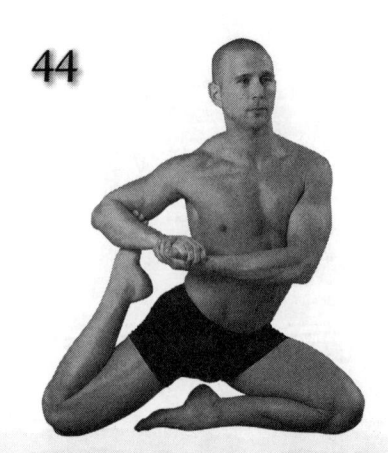

41

42

43

44

PRASARA YOGA: *Flow Beyond Thought*

Repeat the Shinbox Switch one more time to finish in the opposite King Pigeon Pose with your left leg back (45–48).

Drop your foot down and bring your knees together to finish in the last Child's Pose to conclude Flock of Pigeons (49).

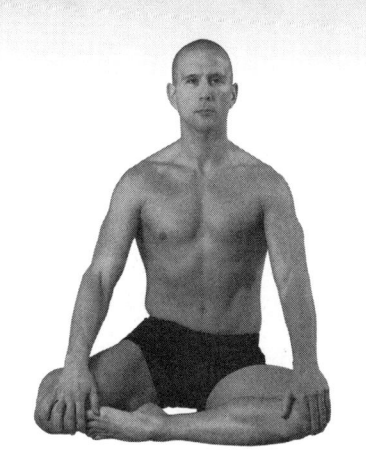

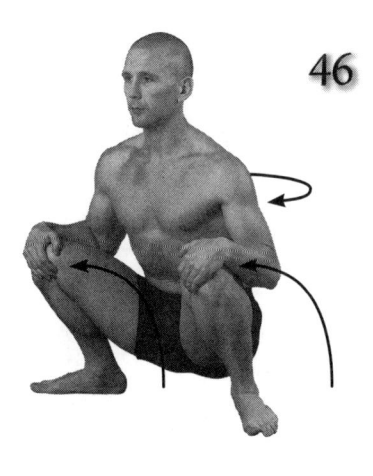

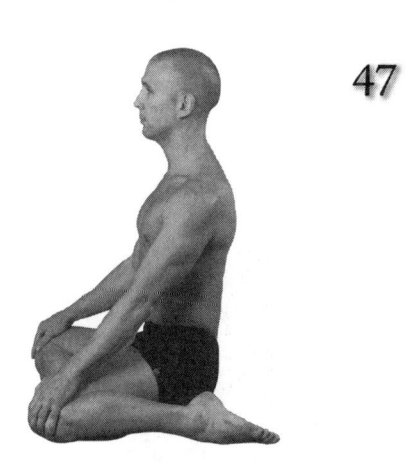

45

46

47

48
(front view)

49

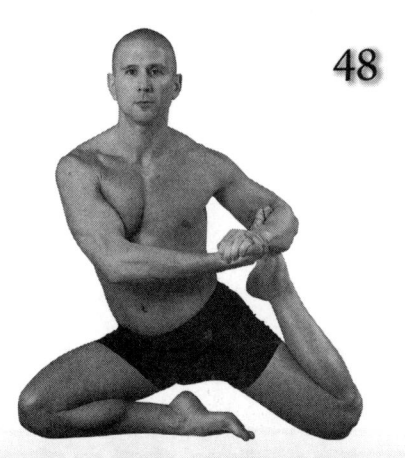

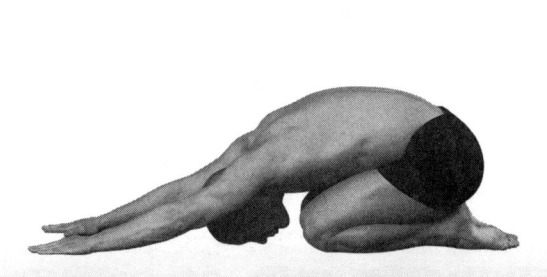

157

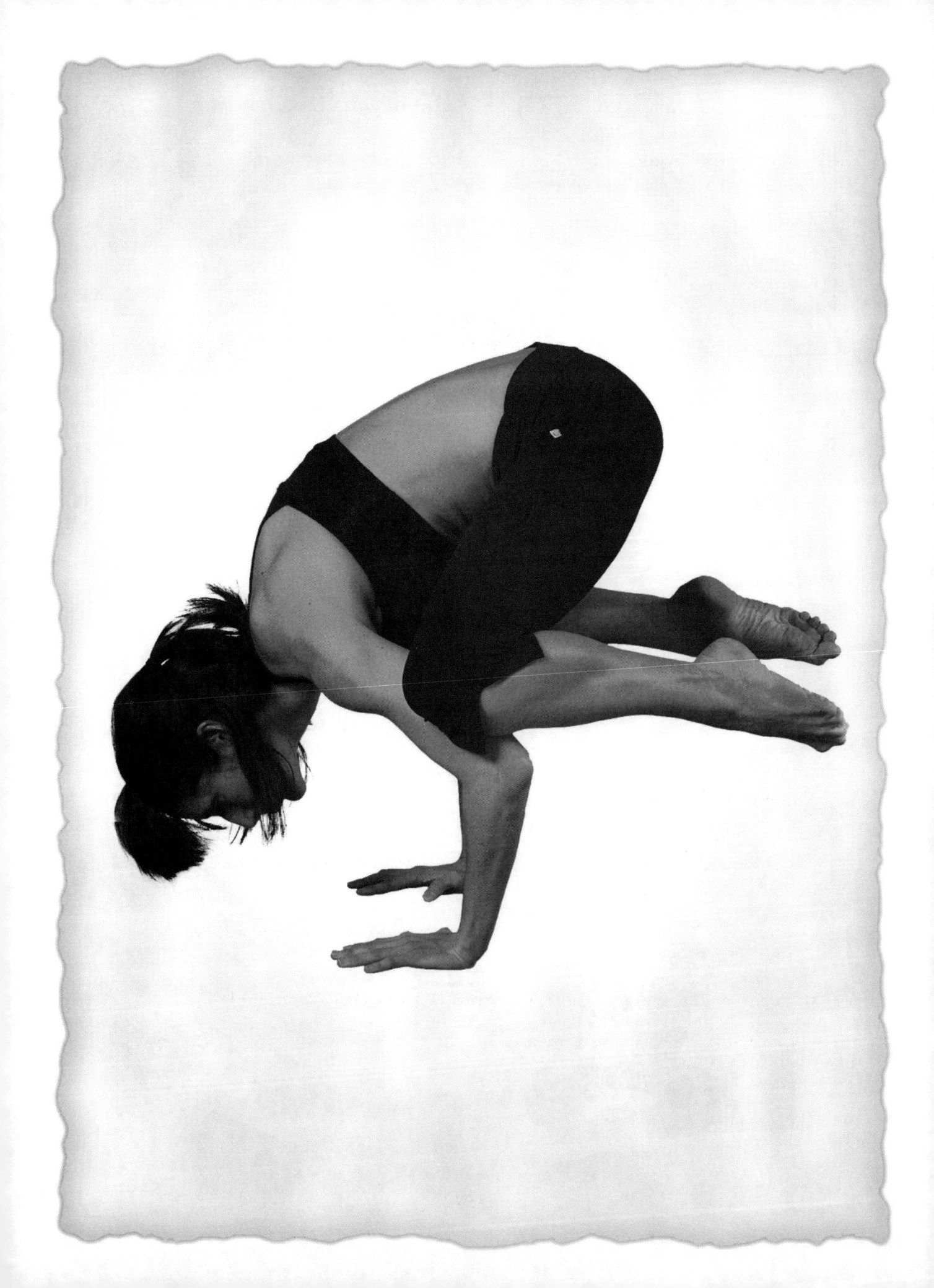

BIBLIOGRAPHY

Alter, Joseph, Ph.D. *The Wrestler's Body: Identity and Ideology in North India*. 1992.

Azar. *APA Monitor.*

Barlow, David. *Anxiety and Its Disorders*. 2nd edition.

Boguk, Nikolay. *Clinical Anatomy of the Lumbar Spine*. 1987.

Bompa, Tudor, Ph.D. *Periodization.*

Boyd, John, Col. *Patterns of Conflict.*

Chek, Paul. "The Inner Unit: A New Frontier In Abdominal Training." *IAAF Technical Quarterly: New Studies in Athletics* (April 1999).

Csikszentmiahlyi, Mihaly. *Creativity: Flow and the Psychology of Discovery and Invention*. New York: Harper Perennial. 1996.

Csikszentmiahlyi, Mihaly. *Finding Flow: The Psychology of Engagement with Everyday Life Basic Books*. reprint edition. April 1998.

Csikszentmiahlyi, Mihaly. *Flow: The Psychology of Optimal Experience*. reprint edition. Harper Perennial. March 13, 1991.

Csikszentmiahlyi, Mihaly. *The Evolving Self*. reprint edition. Harper Perennial. August 3, 1994.

Csikszentmiahlyi, Mihaly. *Flow in Sports*. Human Kinetics Publishers. June 1999.

Damasio, Antonio. *Descartes' Error.*

Dawkins, Richard. *The Selfish Gene.*

DesMaisons, Kathleen. *Potatoes Not Prozac.*

PRASARA YOGA: *Flow Beyond Thought*

Frolov, Vladimir, MD. *Endogenous Respiration.*

Fuller, Buckminster. *Synergetics.* New York: MacMillan. 1975.

Goleman, Daniel. *Emotional Intelligence.* reprint edition. Bantam. June 2, 1997.

Hanna, Thomas. *Somatics: Reawakening the Mind's Control of Movement, Flexibility, and Health.* new ed edition. Da Capo Press. August 3, 2004.

Hearn, Editha. *You Are as Young as Your Spine.* 3rd edition. Bunim & Bannigan Ltd. September 2006.

Ilano, Jarlo. "Combined Movements." RMAX International Forum. June 22, 2004.

Iyengar, B. K. S. *Light on Yoga.* revised edition. Schocken. January 3, 1995.

Jamison, Kay Redfield. *Exuberance: The Passion for Life.* Knopf. September 21, 2004.

Jesse, John. *Wrestling Physical Conditioning Encyclopedia.* Athletic Press. 1970.

Kehoe, Thomas David. *Paul Fitts' Three Stages Involved in Learning a New Skill.* 1997.

Korfist, Chris. "The Foundation." *Intensity Magazine.* Vol. 1, Issue 39, July 9, 2002.

Laban, Rudolf. *Labanotation.*

Laban, Rudolf. *The Mastery of Movement.* Plymouth, UK: Northcote House. 1988.

Lephart, Scott M., and Freddie Fu. *Proprioception and Neuromuscular Control in Joint Stability.*

Levine, Peter. *Healing Trauma: Waking the Tiger.*

Myers, Thomas W. *Anatomy Trains: Myofascial Meridians for Manual and Movement Therapists.* Churchill Livingstone. 2001.

Pert, Candace. *Journal of Immunology.*

Pert, Candace. *Molecules of Emotion.*

Pressfield, Steven. *The War of Art.* reprint edition. Warner Books. April 1, 2003.

Raiport, Grigori MD, Ph.D. *Red Gold: Peak Performance Techniques of the Russian and East German Olympic Victors.* Los Angeles: Jeremy Tarcher Inc. 1988.

Richardson, Jull, Hodges, and Hides. *Therapeutic Exercise for Spinal Segmental Stabilization in Low Back Pain.* 1999.

PRASARA YOGA: *Flow Beyond Thought*

Rothschild, Babette. *The Body Remembers: The Psychophysiology of Trauma and Trauma Treatment.* 1st edition. W. W. Norton & Company. October 15, 2000.

Sapolsky, Robert. *Why Zebras Don't Get Ulcers.*

Siff, Mel, Ph.D. *Facts and Fallacies of Fitness.*

Siff, Mel, Ph.D. *Supertraining.*

Spielman, Ed. *The Spiritual Journey of Joseph Greenstein.*

Soho, Takuan, *The Unfettered Mind.*

Sonnon, Scott. *Big Book of Clubbell Training,* RMAX.tv Productions.

Sonnon, Scott. *Flow-Fighting & the Flow-State Performance Spiral: Peak Performance in Combat Sports.*

Verkhoshansky, Yuri, Ph.D. *Supertraining: Special Strength Training for Sporting Excellence.*

Yessis, Michael, Ph.D. *Secrets of Soviet Sports Fitness & Training.* New York: Arbor House. 1987.

Zatsiorsky, Vladimir, Ph.D. *Science and Practice of Strength Training.*

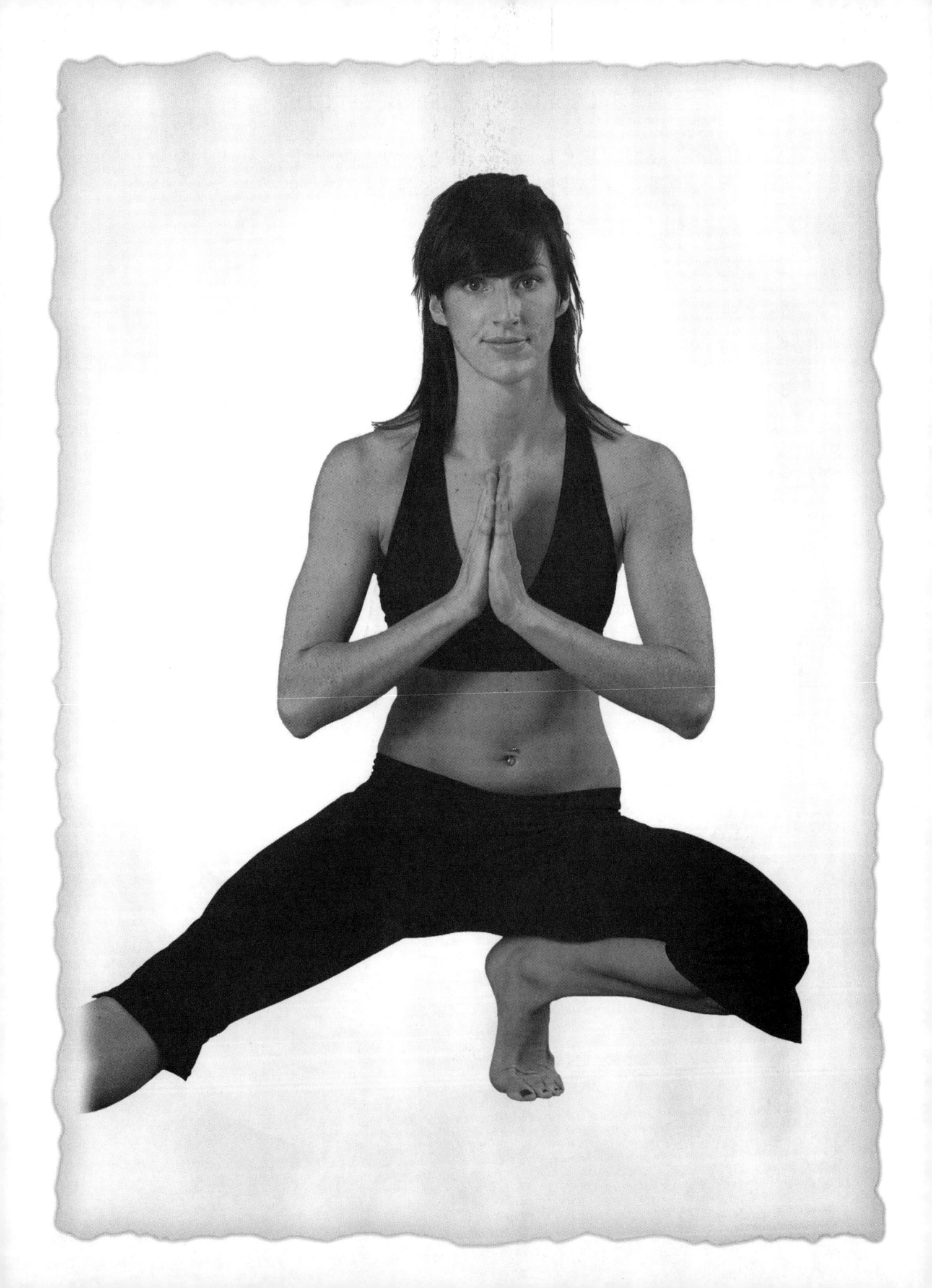